A GOOD DEATH

A GOOD DEATH

An Argument for
Voluntary Euthanasia

RODNEY SYME

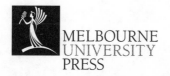

MELBOURNE
UNIVERSITY
PRESS

MELBOURNE UNIVERSITY PRESS
An imprint of Melbourne University Publishing Limited
187 Grattan Street, Carlton, Victoria 3053, Australia
mup-info@unimelb.edu.au
www.mup.com.au

First published 2008
Text © Rodney Syme, 2008
Design and typography © Melbourne University Publishing Ltd 2008

Text design by Phil Campbell
Cover design by Phil Campbell
Typeset by Midland Typesetters, Australia
Printed by Griffin Press, SA

National Library of Australia Cataloguing-in-Publication entry

Syme, Rodney.
    A good death / author, Rodney Syme.
    Carlton, Vic. : Melbourne University Publishing, 2008.

    9780522855036 (pbk.)

    Includes index.
    Bibliography.

    Euthanasia.
    Right to die.
    Assisted suicide.
    Physician and patient.
    Medical ethics.

179.7

FOREWORD

Our felt sense of what is real seems not to include our own death. We doubt the one thing that is not open to any doubt at all.

Sam Harris, *The End of Faith*

'It's not curable. The usual outlook is one to eight years.'

We all know, at one level, that one day we will die; but at another level we don't really, truly, believe it. Most of us, most of the time, don't think about it much. This is probably a healthy thing. You would never enjoy your life if you thought constantly about your death. Yet nearly all of us, unless we die suddenly in a car accident or pass away peacefully in our sleep, will some day be forced to confront the reality of our death: not at some vague, indeterminate time in the future, but soon.

In September 2004 I was forced to confront the reality of my death when I was told I had multiple myeloma, a cancer of the bone marrow, which was, and remains, incurable. People are different: their reactions to this kind of news are different. I did not rail against God, or fate, or ask, 'Why me?' as others have told me they did. I considered it a matter of bad luck, nothing more. I did not even vow, as many do, to fight the cancer, to not 'let this thing beat me'. I accepted, with sadness, that my life, for whatever was left of it, would never again be the same as the one I had known.

But while people react differently to the news that they have an incurable illness, there are also commonalities, as I have found from talking to others who have received a similar diagnosis. One is a wish that our dying will not be painful and protracted; more than dying, we fear what we might have to endure before we die. Another is a wish that we might die with dignity; none of us wants to think we will end our days *sans* speech, *sans* mobility, *sans* sense, being spoon-fed and toileted by our adult children, those same children we once spoon-fed and toileted.

Perhaps the most common reaction is the desire to take *control*. All but the most religious feel this. We are responsible adults. We have autonomy over every aspect of our lives. Why then should we not have autonomy in the matter of the ending of our lives?

We put our affairs in order as much as we can; we write our wills, if we have not already done so; we lie awake at night, planning our funerals. Yet we do these things with the fear that at the end, we will have neither autonomy nor control. The euphemism 'Dying with Dignity' is in fact an accurate description of what most people want.

I am a journalist. I knew Dr Rodney Syme before I became ill. I had interviewed him in the past for articles I had written about what is variously called voluntary euthanasia, medically assisted suicide, dying with dignity legislation. A short time after I received my diagnosis, I contacted Dr Syme. He agreed to meet and talk with me. We met, several times, and after being convinced I was not mentally impaired, was not suffering depression and was not about to take my life at the first opportunity, Dr Syme helped me; he gave me the knowledge I needed to end my life peacefully and painlessly *if and when it became unbearable*. In giving me that knowledge, Dr Syme gave me peace of mind. It is, as he said, good palliative care.

I am aware of my privileged position, that many other people desire what I have. Opinion polls in recent years have shown that the majority of the population—consistently, more than 70 per cent—want the laws changed to allow people to be helped to die. Even religious people want this. A Newspoll in 2007 showed 74 per cent of Australian Catholics would support a doctor 'providing a lethal dose' (not administering) to a person with intolerable and unrelievable suffering.

That is why *A Good Death* is a very necessary book. The proposals in it are not radical. Rodney Syme does not believe in 'euthanasia on demand'. He does not believe that any person who would prefer to submit to God, or fate, in the matter of their dying, should ever feel pressured to do otherwise. His definition of voluntary euthanasia is: 'An action taken by, or at the request of, a rational, fully informed individual, whose intention is to be relieved of intolerable and otherwise unrelievable suffering, that hastens death in a dignified manner'. This is also, despite the many case studies of distressing, painful and difficult end-of-life decisions, ultimately a hopeful book because it carries with it a sense of the inevitability of change: that those individuals who would impose on others—even those who do not share their religious convictions—the unwanted prolongation of life in futile and undignified circumstances will increasingly be seen to be acting invalidly.

The past two centuries have seen in Western societies an enormous expansion of human rights: the abolition of slavery, the ending of child labour, the emancipation of women, universal suffrage and, more recently, the growth of laws banning discrimination on the grounds of race, gender or age. It is an anomaly that, at the beginning of the twenty-first century, we still do not have the right to decide the timing and the manner of our dying.

This is surely a kindness this society, at this stage of its history, owes itself. For as Rodney Syme says, 'A right to live does not include an obligation to do so, under any or every circumstance. It is surely true that we can waive such a right, and this is the basis of our autonomy in end-of-life decisions'.

Pamela Bone

CONTENTS

PREFACE

Voluntary euthanasia, or physician-assisted dying as I prefer to call it, is an intriguing subject to most people. It intrigues because it is about very fundamental matters that many people realise may one day concern them, but which they are reluctant to look at too closely. It also fascinates simply from an intellectual and philosophical level. Most people have a view about it, but without any personal experience of it. When they consider physician-assisted dying, they do so in an abstract and perhaps fearful way. What may be difficult for a non-sufferer in the abstract may however be crystal clear for a sufferer in practice. It is like a person trying to express a view about the game of cricket or baseball, when they have never seen a game and have not read the rules. Moreover, many of the people who write about the subject do so from a theoretical perspective, quoting the views of other 'authorities' who are also quite likely never to have talked in detail with someone who has requested physician-assisted dying. It is also likely that these authorities have never been intimately involved in such assistance. It is a different story for the profound sufferer, who, being at the heart of the matter, can see the issue very clearly. All of the people whom I have helped to die, and discuss in this book, made unequivocal decisions about ending their own lives.

When Steve Guest, dying of oesophageal cancer, rang radio presenter Jon Faine to say that he wanted to end his life, Faine wondered why this could be so, as Steve sounded so rational, as though rational people could not consider ending their lives. Faine had not met Steve, and could not, on radio, visualise his wasting and his exhaustion. How could Faine, at that moment, understand Steve's suffering? When they met, a week later, the absurdity of Faine's earlier comment about rationality was revealed. His subsequent meeting with Steve would have done more than any reading of books or discussions with experts to bring an understanding of these issues. The people who take advantage of physician-assisted dying rarely leave accounts of the process, although fortunately Steve did. Moreover, since in most Western countries voluntary euthanasia is illegal, doctors are extremely loath to talk about their experiences.

And that is exactly why I have written this book—to reveal the context in which these experiences take place, to illuminate the 'black hole' of misunderstanding and ignorance by telling stories from my personal experience of assisting people with intolerable suffering to die with dignity. It is abundantly clear to me that voluntary euthanasia, or physician-assisted dying, is highly dependent on the context of the situation, and it is not easily thoroughly understood by those who have not faced or explored these situations. I believe this understanding of physician-assisted dying is severely hindered by a lack of knowledge in the community of the context in which these decisions are made. Over the past thirty years I have had significant experience of physician-assisted dying in many forms, requested, discussed, denied and assisted. This book is designed to fill a contextual gap in the physician-assisted-dying debate by describing a number of patient–doctor interactions in some depth.

Physician-assisted dying is illegal in all English speaking countries except the State of Oregon in the United States. I know of only one book written by a doctor about his experience, *Dancing with Mister D*, by the Dutch nursing-home physician Bert Keizer.[1] There are occasional short articles in the medical press by doctors describing, usually anonymously, their involvement. Most notable are those by Dr Timothy Quill[2] and Dr Walter Kade.[3] These accounts leave one in no doubt of the profound emotion and difficulty experienced by the doctor, but also in no doubt about the clarity and certainty of their patients. It is this certainty that ultimately allows the doctor to participate. This mirrors my experience—that those not faced with the problem find it extremely confusing, but those dying with intolerable suffering, and who ask for help, can find it a clear, but never easy, decision.

PREFACE

There are a vast number of other books written on this intriguing subject by bystanders: by bioethicists, by legal experts, by theologians, by social researchers and by journalists, who gather opinions and empirical research to form the basis of often very erudite writing and analysis. Much is written by palliative care specialists, but even this output is affected by a mindset that denies the reality of the request, and thus these writers do not go to the heart of the matter, with a complete and open dialogue and final assistance. This lack of an extensive personal medical literature on physician-assisted dying is why it is easy for opponents of the practice to seriously suggest that frail and disabled people will be persuaded to request assistance in dying against their will, and even more bizarrely, that they will be given assistance, against their will. It just does not happen. People simply do not ask for help to die because someone else thinks it is a good idea. This book has been written to illuminate just what does happen. More specifically, it reveals what happens when assistance in dying must be covert, and the difficulties that accompany practice in such circumstances.

Because I am telling the stories of a number of my patients, whose names have been changed so as not to disclose their identities, this book is inevitably also about me. It is not my intention that it should be so, but it is unavoidable. I must be the voice who speaks on behalf of each of these people, because they can no longer speak for themselves. I have approached each person in an open fashion, willing to listen, learn and assess. I have never attempted to impose my position as may occur in palliative care, where the starting position does not include deliberate ending of life, even if this is requested by the patient. Each request has a context that is developed through a dialogue between the suffering individual and myself, and the story cannot be told without my contribution. This is my honest account of some of my experience. This has been an extremely difficult book to write because it exposes me to the possibility of heavy criticism, and the possibility of prosecution. Some of these particular stories have been chosen because these people have left significant statements of their views, which enhance the stories. Together, perhaps, the two voices that are missing in this debate (those who are suffering in dying and their doctors) will be better understood.

Because this is a personal story, it is appropriate to tell a little about myself. I was born in 1935 into a well-off medical family, part of the Melbourne establishment. I attended an Anglican (Protestant) private school, where the emphasis seemed to be on humanist enlightenment values, with an exposure to the life of Christ, rather than on biblical dogma. A subsequent exposure to scientific disciplines made it impossible to believe in a resurrection and an after-life, and a study of Darwin and genetics made the necessity for God irrelevant. In terms of my beliefs, I would call myself a Christian humanist. Some might see this as an oxymoron, but I do recognise that my values have been influenced by my education and life in the Western (Christian) tradition. However, this is more an influence of the teachings attributed to Jesus than by the Christian religion as practised by most of its churches. I do not accept the resurrection, but I am impressed by the values of compassion, tolerance and inclusivity exhibited by Jesus. The very same values may well have been derived without any knowledge of Christ, but I cannot deny that influence.

History has been a lifelong passion, and has confirmed the banal effects of organised religion. These effects are certainly evident in the opposition to physician-assisted dying, which seeks to impose a particular view on all. Gradually my experiences in medicine led me to a position where my conscience, formed by these influences, simply would not let me ignore the requests for assistance made by people with intense suffering.

Readers will note that I rarely use the word 'patient' to describe the people who have sought my advice. This is deliberate. The word 'patient' is commonly used to describe a person who seeks advice from a doctor, or who is ill and undergoing treatment. However, the application of this term to a person may subtly alter the way they see themselves, and the way they are treated by their doctors, nurses and carers. It categorises them as being in a dependent role, and, in a subtle way, they tend to lose their autonomy. The doctor is perceived as being superior and as dictating the relationship, and as a person who directs rather than advises. Thus, the use of this word to describe terminally or hopelessly ill people significantly affects the relationship between the doctor and that person. They become a patient with a disease who needs medical treatment, rather than an individual who is suffering and who has individual needs. As Eric Cassel wrote, in his classic essay on *Diagnosing Suffering*,[4] 'suffering is an affliction of the person, not the body'. The most important of those needs is to be understood as a whole person, and for consideration to be given to the totality of their suffering, not just their obvious medical symptoms. Palliative care understands this, and this is why it is usually very successful in caring for dying people.

I have also deliberately avoided discussing the role of religion in this matter. It has a very significant influence in why we are where we are, but no place in where we ought to go. Discussion of its general impact is not relevant to a discussion of the context of individual deaths. It is the subject of a book in its own right.

In my opinion, there is a conspiracy of a benevolent kind between medicine, the law, the prosecuting authorities and government to hide the reality that physician–assisted deaths do happen covertly in homes, in hospices and in hospitals. This conspiracy is, of course, not in any sense organised. That reality is simply quietly acknowledged and left undisturbed, and that is why doctors are not prosecuted for assisting people to die. In the past, I had hoped it would protect me, and it has. Covert practice, however, no matter how well intentioned, is not appropriate.

The law as it stands is not clear in relation to medical practice at the end of life. Yet the possibility of its application causes confusion and fear to govern most medical decisions at the end of life, and patients suffer as a result. There is an urgent need for this crucial issue to be referred to a law reform commission to advise government on legislative change with appropriate safeguards.

Recently in Australia, the debate on voluntary euthanasia was side-tracked by the suicide of an 80-year-old Perth woman, Lisette Nigot. The media reported that she was 'well' and that her suicide note stated, 'I want to end it before it gets bad'. The impression was that she was 'tired of life' and did not have any particular suffering. She was a very mature individual who was not depressed in any way. On the face of it, this seemed to be a pre-emptive act to prevent problems in the future as much as a release from current boredom. These are not indications for physician-assisted dying in any current or proposed legislation. Whatever one may think of the philosophical argument that any person has the right to end their life when they determine, this has nothing to do with the argument for the legislation of medical assistance for the relief of intolerable and unrelievable suffering. It is simply not a part of any serious legislative proposal.

Most of this book was written before I met Steve Guest. That meeting was influential in changing the direction of the book from a focus on the context around end-of-life decisions to a more direct legal challenge to the status quo. Although I did not set out to do so, I believe this book also enunciates a challenge to palliative care. Through the analysis of the stories of these dying people, a picture of the deficiencies of palliative care emerges. Some in palliative care are aware of this. The challenge is to expand palliative care to truly respect autonomy and adequately relieve suffering. It can be done.

I hope this book leads to change. It reveals a lot about intention, and about suffering, about dignity, about control, about respect and about choice. These things matter to us all, and that is ultimately why I am telling this story.

Rodney Syme

ACKNOWLEDGEMENTS

This has not been an easy book to write. There have been many occasions when I seriously questioned what I was doing. I realised that I was exposing myself to some legal risk. As time went on I began to feel that this was not as great as I had first feared. But I was also exposing myself, my values and beliefs, my fears and my weakness, to public scrutiny. I was also exposing my family to risk. Without the tremendous support of my wife Meg and my children Robin, Bruce and Megan I would not have completed the task. Moreover, they were a constant sounding board for ideas and criticism, and reassurance that I was not off my rocker. They have all taught me so much throughout my life.

My ideas on suffering at the end of life have been formed by conversations with many courageous people over thirty years. It is they who have taught me, and it has been a privilege to help them in some way. My education in bioethics owes most to Helga Kuhse and Peter Singer, who have been a profound help in this area.

It has been difficult to discuss these matters with other doctors, and my major source of medical assistance has come from doctors I have met through the World Federation of Right to Die Societies. These wonderful men—Aycke Smook, Michael Irwin, Richard MacDonald and Stanley Terman in particular—have all faced the same problems as I, and have been free with their support and advice in coping with them.

I have been closely associated over the past seventeen years with Dying With Dignity Victoria (previously the Voluntary Euthanasia Society of Victoria). Many wonderful colleagues on the committee of management and in the organisation generally deserve recognition for their unrealised contributions to this book. I particularly thank the Executive Officers I have worked with—Kay Koetsier, Lindy Boyd and Rowena Moore.

I also thank friends in the South Australian Voluntary Euthanasia Society, Mary Gallnor and Frances Coombe, who have been close advisers.

Jane Edwards and Michael Craig have been of tremendous help in reading and advising on the manuscript. It is not their fault if the text retains some of my stubborn idiosyncracies.

Finally, I thank all those at Melbourne University Publishing who have been so helpful in polishing the manuscript and making it readable, particularly Sybil Nolan, Elisa Berg and Valina Rainer. And finally I thank Pamela Bone for opening the door for me at MUP.

1

EPIPHANY

'There are two or three pain syndromes that are particularly difficult for us to treat, nerve pain, bone pain, and pain that is largely comprised of suffering in the psychological sphere.'
Michael Ashby, Professor of Palliative Care, Monash University

It was a lovely autumn day in Melbourne. Those who know Melbourne will appreciate how peaceful this environment can be. The days are warm and mild, with blue skies and a gentle breeze. But I was not at peace. I was about to visit a woman suffering from secondary cancer in her spine. Despite every effort by me and my colleagues, Betty's life was becoming a viciously painful nightmare. As I approached the stairs leading to her room, I heard her screams of anguish as the nurses tried to place her on a bed-pan.

This was uncharted territory for me. I was forty years old and well into a medical career as a specialist urologist. I had been a doctor for fifteen years, yet I had never had the responsibility for, and close contact with, a terminally ill person with very severe escalating pain and suffering. My experience had been entirely in hospitals, a passing parade of people, most of whom were treated and got better. A small number had died but usually in acute circumstances. I had not been responsible for slowly dying patients.

In those days, most people with terminal illness were dealt with by their general practitioner or by physicians specialising in terminal illness. For the first time in my career, I came face to face with intolerable and unrelievable suffering which I had the responsibility to manage. I was uneducated and ill-prepared to do so. I summoned all possible support from my colleagues but to no avail. A sense of helplessness, shame and guilt accompanied me on my daily visits. I was determined not to abandon Betty by not visiting, and I would sit in my car outside the hospital whilst I summoned up the courage to go into the ward, often to be met by her cries of pain. It is extremely difficult to face another human being whom you know has intolerable suffering for which you have no answer. No wonder many palliative care workers suffer 'burn out'. My emotional distress was considerable, but nothing compared to Betty's physical and emotional anguish, and that of her family. Her suffering was so severe, hastening her death was essentially the only way to relieve her suffering. She did not ask for this and I cannot remember whether this thought crossed my mind at that time. But it certainly did over the succeeding months as I thought deeply about this experience.

In 1972, I had removed Betty's right kidney, which contained a large cancer. She was a 52-year-old, happily married woman with two children. I was pleased at the outcome of this difficult operation, as she remained well for two years and appeared to be cured. Unfortunately, unknown to me, the cancer had already spread to others parts of her body. Betty returned in 1974, complaining of severe pain in her lower back. Investigation showed that the cancer had spread into her upper lumbar vertebrae, causing collapse of the bone. Very soon, she was also experiencing very severe, at times excruciating pain radiating into her legs and difficulty with urination, due to pressure on her spinal cord and nerves. Betty was clearly incurably ill, with severe bone pain and nerve pain. After I explained the implications of the X-ray findings, she realised the gravity of her situation. She now fulfilled Professor Ashby's three difficult pain conditions—bone pain, nerve pain and psychological pain. She realised that little could be done by way of relief, and that the pain would continue and probably increase until she died. She had an incurable illness, was arguably terminally ill, meaning that her death could be anticipated within say six months. She was not in the imminently dying phase of a terminal illness.

I tried desperately to relieve her pain, but there was then no effective chemotherapy for kidney cancer. I arranged for a neurosurgeon to operate on her spine in an attempt to relieve the pressure on the nerves, but the rich blood supply and extent of the cancer prevented any benefit. The pain from kidney cancer may sometimes be reduced, or palliated, by radiotherapy, but a course of this treatment provided no relief. Nerve pain can sometimes be relieved by blocking or dividing the affected nerves above the point of irritation. In Betty's case, it would have involved a further operation to divide the pain-conducting fibres in the spinal cord on both sides in the upper chest region, above the point of involvement by the cancer, rendering her totally insensitive in the lower half of the body and destroying bladder and bowel function. This was not an acceptable procedure for a person with a relatively short life expectancy. Palliative care was not yet a reality in Melbourne in 1974, and there were, to my knowledge, only two doctors specialising in difficult pain management. A consultation between one of them and Betty unsurprisingly indicated that the only 'effective' therapy was narcotic drugs (usually morphine) to diminish both the constant bone pain and the more severe episodic nerve (neuropathic) pain.

Constant pain can be reasonably well relieved by narcotics, but severe episodic pain is another matter. Betty's pain was continually present, but with any movement involving the spine, as in turning in bed, changing position or getting onto a bed-pan, excruciating 'incident' pain would occur. This pain was due to acute nerve pressure, exactly as when your dentist drills into an unanaesthetised nerve in your tooth. It was so sudden and severe that it could not be relieved even by regular injections of morphine. Such a pain essentially requires a deep anaesthetic for control. In 1974 the idea of delivering continuous high dose analgesics and sedatives to control such pain was unknown. In the climate of those times, doctors and nurses (and to a lesser extent still today) were fearful that if they delivered large doses of narcotics, which could hasten death through their side-effects, they might be hauled before the law. They did not understand that, in this situation, the dose required is the dose that works, not the dose that is safe. In such situations it needs only one person with a moral objection to hastening death in any circumstances to make an official complaint for a criminal or Medical Board investigation to become a reality. This principle of pain palliation in terminal situations is now more widely understood, but was barely appreciated then. The possibility of complaint was a finite reality, and while it is less so today, many doctors and nurses who lack experience are still inhibited by the law from delivering adequate pain relief. One eminent doctor has pointed out the difficulties for medical practitioners in what should be a commonsense treatment situation: 'the optimal treatment of pain and adverse effects of analgesics requires aggressive use of controlled substances (opioids and barbiturates), potentially raising fears of regulatory scrutiny, or the disapproval of professional colleagues'.[1] This fear and uncertainty exists, despite the Guidelines of the American Geriatrics Society that say 'it is the responsibility of physicians to relieve pain, especially when the prognosis is poor; pain relief may be the most important thing physicians can offer their patients'.[2]

Betty's suffering continued unabated over two months of absolute misery. Her agony was extreme and I was powerless to do anything about it, except to exhort the nurses to give larger and more frequent doses of morphine. Despite my orders, the nurses were reluctant to do so. Thinking about this over the next few months, I realised that a doctor in this situation may need to show leadership and not only prescribe the appropriate doses, but also personally administer them. But at that time, I didn't know that.

Betty's pain could be relieved only by massive—virtually anaesthetic—doses of morphine, rendering her insensitive to any feeling at all. The amount of morphine required to even partially relieve her pain would have caused respiratory depression and hastened her death. Her death was not imminent, but the measures necessary for the relief of her agony would make it so.

In 1974, medical assistance in dying (euthanasia) was not a common subject of media or even medical discussion. It had not been part of my undergraduate or postgraduate education. It only became a subject of serious medical and public debate in 1973 when a Dutch GP hastened the death of her mother. I knew little about this subject, and was therefore not 'open' to any signals that Betty or her family may have sent. She did not ever ask me to hasten her death. Her husband once asked me 'if there was something more that I could do'; I did not recognise that as a signal to begin a dialogue about hastening death (if indeed it was), but today I would certainly do so. Patients, and their relatives on their behalf, do not often directly broach the question of a hastened death, as they realise that they are asking a highly charged question. Moreover, if the patient or her family raise the question in the presence of others (such as nurses), it only makes the doctor's position more difficult. Doctors need to be alert to the subtle signals that indicate a particular person is ready to develop a dialogue about their future. In 1974, I would have almost certainly 'taken refuge' behind the law, which makes such dialogue difficult and often pointless unless circumstances are favourable, such as a home situation where privacy is secure. I was simply not prepared by experience, understanding or education to be open to such a signal, even though I was now acutely aware that a society that would not allow an animal to suffer such pain would allow a sentient human being to do so.

When Betty's husband asked if she could be moved to another hospital closer to her home to allow easier visiting, I have to admit that I readily agreed and felt relieved of a huge burden as she passed out of my care.

Betty's suffering caused me great anguish. As a urologist, I was accustomed to achieving a high degree of success in dealing with my patients' problems. It had been rare for me to be exposed to the management of this stage of a terminal illness. I was not aware, from personal experience, of the reality of dying of cancer. This seminal experience started a singular journey as I gradually learnt more of this reality over the next thirty years, both from experience and from close study of the palliative care literature. There I found that physical symptoms in the person in the terminal phase of disease are associated with increasing distress, as well as major depression and anxiety; severe pain that is inadequately controlled and poorly tolerated has been associated with suicide in cancer patients. In addition the burden of illness is borne by family members who may also experience distress and poor health, financial problems, and disruption to their work lives.[3]

Michael Ashby, Professor of Palliative Care at Melbourne's Monash University, specifically defined problematic pain as *nerve pain, bone pain, and pain that is largely comprised of suffering in the psychological sphere* (my italics).[4] Betty had all these phenomena, and I felt an enormous sense of failure as I had been unable to have any impact on her problem. My reaction was wrong but natural because there was almost nothing that anybody could have done in these circumstances at that time.

As I thought about this experience, my guilt and shame were replaced by anger and frustration. I realised that my inability to help Betty more effectively was not because of any lack of caring or compassion on my part. It was because the law inhibited a dialogue of any substance to develop between us about alternative ways of treatment to relieve her of this profound and intolerable suffering. It is cruel to commence a dialogue that raises the hope and spirits of a patient if one does not have any inclination, or more importantly, any ability to take that dialogue to a conclusion. Why did the law prevent such humane assistance? Was it the religion behind the origins of our Western law that was responsible? The Catholic Church was implacably opposed to hastening death in order to relieve suffering, and claimed salvific value in suffering while dying.[5]

I quickly realised that I would not have allowed myself to suffer as Betty had suffered. I am absolutely certain that in the same circumstances I would have taken the opportunity to end my own life. Of course, as a doctor, I could very easily do this. First, I had knowledge about pathology and disease that is essential to understanding just how my illness would progress. Second, I had knowledge about pharmacology and drugs that would allow me to choose a drug or combination of drugs that would reliably end my life with dignity and security. Third, I had access to drugs or to helpful colleagues for the prescription of the necessary drugs. Therefore, when my time came, I would be all right. I would have control. Additionally, on reflection, I would not have accepted such appalling unrelieved suffering for one of my family.

However, I could not help thinking how grossly unfair this was for others who did not have my advantages as a doctor. Many people with terminal illness do take their own lives in order to end their suffering, but, lacking knowledge and opportunity, do so in the most horrific circumstances. Shooting, hanging, cutting of wrists or throat, jumping from heights, or in front of trains, deliberate motor accidents or gassing and corrosive poisoning are the commonly employed methods and often occur without discussion with relatives, leaving an appalling and indelible memory. Such lonely deaths are rarely if ever discussed with the family and leave a savage legacy of psychological pain for those left behind.

I could have forgotten this incident—with any luck I would have been unlikely to meet such a circumstance again, and to date have not. But I could not dismiss it—why I do not know, except that I sensed that there was something seriously wrong with our law and society that could allow such suffering. Gradually, I came to the firm conclusion that people with hopeless and incurable illness should have the right to assistance to end their lives if their suffering is unrelievable and intolerable. I also realised that it was wrong to feel guilt and shame at being unable to help patients in this situation, for it was not I who was at fault but the law that created this situation. I also gradually realised, over the following years, however, that I would continue to feel diminished if I did not try to do something to help such people in the future. It would have weighed too heavily on my conscience to do otherwise.

2

THE JOURNEY BEGINS

'The Parliament recognizes that it is desirable to ensure that dying patients receive maximum relief from pain and suffering.'
Preamble to the *Victorian Medical Treatment Act, 1988*

The Australian Medical Association supports 'doctors whose primary intent is to relieve the suffering and distress of terminally ill patients, in accordance with the patient's wishes and interests, even though a foreseen consequence is the hastening of death'.
AMA Federal Assembly, May 2002

I often conduct workshops for Dying with Dignity Victoria, a law reform organisation, to explain how people can prepare to achieve a peaceful and dignified death. One important action is to appoint an agent (medical enduring power of attorney) to make medical decisions on your behalf if you become mentally incompetent to make your own decisions. Personal friendship and family relationship can make such decisions difficult and emotional, since neither friend nor family wants to lose their loved one. Thus such an agent must be someone you trust implicitly, but also someone with the understanding and courage to carry out your choices. That agent must also fully understand the life views and treatment choices of their appointer, and not act unless it is absolutely clear that they are fulfilling those wishes. They must be clearly acting in the expressed best interests of that person, and that means the best interests as explained and not as presumed. This requires excellent levels of communication.

I had known Ken, a member of my wife's family, for a long time and we had discussed end-of-life matters on many occasions. I knew him and his views extremely well. I had no doubt about his attitude to prolonging a life of suffering, and that he agreed with the philosophy of hastening death to relieve intolerable suffering. He had suffered a number of health problems, and had battled on with them, but as he grew older, his heart began to fail. He became increasingly breathless and was treated in hospital on several occasions for crises due to severe heart failure—his heart problems were steadily becoming worse.

In 1975, Ken was again admitted to hospital with a further episode of very severe heart failure, and his heart was massively enlarged. His breathing distress was extreme and he had shown no improvement with treatment. His family was extremely concerned at his distress and asked me to see him. He was in a hospital where I treated some of my own patients, so I visited him that afternoon.

I was appalled by his situation. He was blue in the face due to lack of oxygen in his blood despite breathing pure oxygen through a mask, and his difficulty in breathing was as bad as anything I had ever seen. He was receiving maximal therapy but without any response.

Ken was in the last stage of dying of heart failure. Between heaving breaths, he quietly gasped, 'Help me!'

It was impossible to have any conversation with him, because he could barely breathe, let alone speak. I could not discuss what exact form of help he wanted, or clarify his request in more explicit terms, and his family was not present to consult. Yet it was clear that he was dying of heart failure, and from our previous dialogue I knew that this was exactly the suffering he wanted to avoid. I had not come to visit him with the intention of helping him to die, but it was crystal clear that this was the only way his suffering would be relieved and was now the decision I had to make. I could not turn my back on his suffering and simply walk away.

I was not his treating doctor, but that doctor had written an order for a large dose of morphine for the relief of respiratory distress. This was exactly what he needed now but the nurses were not responding, either through fear or ignorance, to his need. Strict medical protocol meant that I should have rung his doctor to discuss the matter of urgent relief of his distress, but this was a medical emergency of no less importance than if he was dying but could be saved. Palliative care expert Declan Walsh said, 'It is unacceptable to allow patients to die with unrelieved respiratory distress. Drug doses should be increased as required for this purpose, even at the risk of hastening death from CNS (central nervous system) depression'.[1] There was no time for medical niceties. I could not waste time tracking down Ken's doctor, and perhaps entering a protracted debate and ending up with an inadequate response.

My mind went back to Betty, my patient in this same hospital, and the reluctance of the nurses to give large doses of narcotic that might hasten death while relieving suffering. I determined to give the injection of morphine myself and asked the nurse to draw up the ordered dose. I gave it to Ken intravenously, for rapid and maximal effect, and recall his almost immediate relief and his mumbled thanks. He passed into a coma as the dose of morphine suppressed respiratory drive and slowed his respiration, the direct effect of the injection. His suffering relieved, he remained asleep until he died about two hours later.

His suffering had been palliated and his family was extremely grateful. I had provided assistance in hastening Ken's death by a large intravenous dose of morphine. Without the injection, he still would have died, but only after some hours of the most appalling and prolonged breathlessness, and the extreme anxiety, bordering on terror, of not knowing whether his next gasp would be his last. I gave him that injection in order to provide maximal palliation of his terminal suffering from gross breathlessness due to cardiac failure. I could not only foresee that this action could hasten his death, but knew that it was extremely likely that it would do so. Was there an explicit detailed request to do so? Perhaps not, but he was in no condition to express more than the simplest request, which he did. In my opinion, he requested it in an oblique way, and I believed that it was in his best interests, as he had previously expressed them to me, to relieve his suffering. My primary intent was immediate palliation, but to be honest I had a secondary intention of bringing his suffering to a final end. That could occur only through his death. His suffering would simply continue until he died. He would not have wanted to wake again to return to the hell from which he had mercifully escaped.

Reflecting on this episode, I am comforted by the words of respiratory specialist Dr Martin Cohen who observed that 'breathlessness however is probably an even more distressing symptom than severe pain'[2] and of other experts who tell us that 'existing methods to control dyspnoea [breathlessness] are ineffective'.[3]

Most discussion of suffering in terminal illness focuses on cancer patients. An editorial from the *British Medical Journal* in 1998 puts the suffering of chronic heart failure in perspective:

> Quality of life in chronic heart failure is poor, and discomfort and distress often worse than in cancer ... People who had died from heart disease, including heart failure, had experienced a wide range of symptoms, often distressing and often lasting more than six months. In addition to dyspnoea, pain, nausea, constipation and low mood were common and poorly controlled. At least one in six had symptoms as severe as those with cancer managed in hospices or by palliative care services.[4]

Other researchers investigating communication and choice in dying from heart disease found that 54 per cent died non-acute deaths in hospital. Forty per cent of patients and 43 per cent of carers felt they had not had enough choice in where they had died. Twenty-three per cent of the patients had expressed a wish to die sooner.[5]

I could have given Ken a smaller dose of morphine by a less rapidly absorbed route, with less risk of hastening death, but which would have been less effective in providing relief. That option would have prolonged Ken's inevitable dying with the certainty of his once again finding himself in exactly the same distress from which he had temporarily escaped. To me, this is a cruel and futile approach, which would be done to protect the legal and perhaps moral interests of the doctor rather than the best interests of the suffering person.

What is the intention of a doctor who administers a large intravenous dose of morphine? This is a complex question, which may be difficult to answer accurately. It is certainly an action taken with the primary intention of relieving suffering. I did not want Ken to die. However, doctors, other carers and families, may also accept that death is not only a foreseen consequence of the injection, but regard it as a welcome consequence. Dr Marcia Angell, editor of one of America's most prestigious medical journals, made this comment:

> Just as family members often feel a sense of relief along with their grief when such patients finally die, so doctors often wish both to ease suffering and to hasten death. The balance of those desires may vary from hour to hour, depending on the patient's condition ... If all attempts at palliation fail, as they sometimes do, then the hope for an easier death may give way to the hope for a faster one. That is, the intent can shift.[6]

Because the suffering will be a recurring problem until death occurs, the doctor may agree that it is in his patient's best interests to die quickly rather than slowly, and, thus, may intend to hasten death while also relieving suffering. The doctor's decision is certainly made easier and more ethical by prior discussion as to the patient's views. Clearly, any intention to hasten death is secondary to the intention to relieve suffering. The intention to hasten death does not exist at all without the concurrent need to aggressively relieve the suffering. For my own part I had hoped more than intended that the injection would hasten Ken's death. This was another seminal moment when I first crossed the Rubicon, the fine line that divides traditional medical practice from the grey area of hastening death. The line is sometimes so fine as to be invisible. Marcia Angell again:

> It is absurd to imagine that doctors could be innocent at one hour, but deserving 20 years in prison in the next, simply because the desired outcome of treatment changed. What is important is whether doctors are doing their utmost to ease suffering in accord with their patient's wishes.[7]

The Council of Judicial and Ethical Affairs of the American Medical Association agrees, stating, 'The ethical distinction between providing palliative care that may have fatal side effects and providing euthanasia is subtle because in both cases the action that caused death is performed with the purpose of relieving suffering'.[8]

The courts recognise this and, as a result, actions of this sort are not the subject of criminal charges. The Australian Medical Association (AMA) supports 'doctors whose primary intent is to relieve the suffering and distress of terminally ill patients, in accordance with the patients' wishes and interests, even though a foreseen secondary consequence is the hastening of death'.[9]

There will be an investigation only if a relative or a carer takes exception to the suddenness of the death. In this case, Ken accepted death as a consequence of relief of suffering, as did his family.

Does it occur to other doctors in this situation, as it did to me, that their injection might hasten death? Of course it does, and they have to decide what dose to give, how to give it, and what its effects will be. If a doctor knows that the necessary treatment will hasten death, then his decision to administer a large dose in a particular way because he knows it to be in the person's best interest is a conscious decision to hasten death. It may also be his intention to honour this person's request while relieving suffering. These two intentions are inextricably linked. I personally find it impossible not to consider both questions when confronted by such dilemmas, and find it extraordinary that some doctors can say they can contemplate these actions with no intention to hasten death. It may be helpful to their conscience but to me it seems a remarkable feat of rationalisation.

The use of morphine by doctors to ease the final anguish, or hasten their death as the case may be, has a long tradition, almost certainly dating to the discovery of the effects of this wonderful drug. I was reminded of this by the following passage from *The Lunar Men*, describing the death of the great English potter and porcelain maker Josiah Wedgwood, treated by his very great friend Dr Erasmus Darwin (grandfather of the celebrated Charles) more than 200 years ago.

> Darwin had kept his friend well enough to say goodbye to his family, but he had given him a private supply of laudanum [extract of morphine]. On 2 January 1795 Wedgwood told Sally and Susannah not to come in as he was sure he would sleep soundly all night. Next morning, they found his room locked from the inside. The carpenter came running with a ladder, and climbed in through the window to find him lying dead.[10]

Morphine as a drug to hasten death is a crude and unreliable option. It does produce respiratory depression, but the dose required is unpredictable and depends very much on prior usage. It works well when there is already respiratory difficulty and is totally justifiable as palliation. It may also work well when a person is already very close to death. It is, of course, hard to justify when there is no pain, and it is a poor drug for confusion, delirium or terror. Despite this, it is widely used by doctors because it is 'safe' for them to prescribe it.

The use of morphine, often in increasingly large doses with cumulative effect, to relieve respiratory distress or very severe pain in a way that hastens death has been excised from the debate about physician-assisted dying. Because the death is gradual, it can be argued that the death was due to the disease and not the treatment, or that the treatment was necessary. One can also argue that the death was not explicitly hastened, and the intention of the doctor was not clear and cannot be determined. His intention is what he says it is.

Nevertheless, there is no doubt that treatment that hastens death with the primary intention of relieving suffering by large doses of narcotics is as old as medicine itself, and is certainly a common practice. In a survey of Australian surgeons, 36 per cent reported that they had 'for the purpose of relieving a patient's suffering, given drugs in doses greater than those required to relieve symptoms, with the intention of hastening death'.[11] If it is an action, taken at the request of a person whose intention is to be relieved of suffering, that hastens death in a dignified manner, then I believe it can be described as an act of voluntary euthanasia in principle.

My assistance to Ken fell neatly into the AMA pronouncement expressed lucidly twenty-seven years later. Thus, such actions have been quarantined from the debate about euthanasia, and are not regarded as representing euthanasia by the AMA, prosecutorial authorities and opponents of physician-assisted dying. This is due to the application of the rule of 'double effect', which states that if an action may have two consequences, one good and the other bad, then it is morally acceptable to carry out that action, provided the bad action was not intended, but merely foreseen. This has religious origins, being first expressed by St Thomas Aquinas in the thirteenth century to resolve some difficult moral dilemmas. It achieved legal and medical significance when Justice Devlin (later Lord Devlin) in the UK in 1957 determined that a doctor could use narcotics to relieve his patient's severe pain, even though the foreseen but unintended consequence was to cause or hasten death (*R v. Adams*). Apart from self-defence, it is only in a medical context that a person is protected from the foreseen consequences of an act that causes death. The problem is that it is extremely difficult, if not impossible, to determine the doctor's intention. In these situations, there is always a prima facie case for the use of the medication. The doctor clearly has the primary intention to relieve suffering, but does he have a secondary intention to hasten death? It does not seem clear whether the law concerns itself with secondary intention.

From a medical point of view, such matters of intention are not so simple. Dr Timothy Quill, an experienced palliative care physician, says that 'Multi-layered intentions are present in most, if not all, end-of-life decisions', and also:

> If we do not acknowledge the inescapable multiplicity of intentions in most double-effect situations, physicians may retreat from aggressive palliative treatment out of fear of crossing the allegedly bright line between allowing patients to die and causing their death. Our current ethical thinking and legal prohibitions reinforce self-deception, secrecy, isolation and abandonment when the exact opposite is needed.[12]

Dr Quill's comment on aggressive palliative treatment is illuminating. Are there two forms of palliative care—one normal and one aggressive? If so, what is meant by 'aggressive' palliative care if it is not palliative care that hastens death while relieving suffering? There seems to be some hypocrisy in the approach taken by the medical profession and condoned by prosecutorial authorities. Although medical actions are commonly closely associated with the timing and manner of death, there is no specific legislation that deals with this difficult area. Doctors are left in uncertainty as to the boundaries of practice, and their patients are worse off as a result.

I have described Ken's last major illness event, but he did have other life-threatening events from heart failure over a few years. He recovered from those events to live tolerably well until the next crisis. This is the typical trajectory of many non-cancer illnesses, particularly chronic cardiac and respiratory conditions. It is quite different from the more predictable, usually progressive, and usually shorter trajectory of cancer, such as we saw with Betty, although with some cancers, successful chemotherapy can produce long remissions after symptomatic relapses.

Although Ken's death was medically and legally sanctioned, was it a 'good death'? It could be described as a 'wild death', a term to denote an unprepared death without peace and in undesirable contexts, especially in the midst of futile attempts to prolong life.[13] When I treated Ken he was dying, but he was dying badly. Would the term 'dysthanasia' be appropriate here (*dys* is the Greek root for *bad* and *thanatos* for *death*)? I think it would, and many people face similar circumstances at the end of their lives. Would compulsory or non-voluntary dysthanasia be an appropriate description for his situation? I think it would, because society imposed this dying on Ken against his express wish—the same society that denied his right to voluntary euthanasia.

Ken did not have the opportunity to say goodbye to his family, he could not make an explicit decision to hasten his death, and he may have wanted his death to come sooner rather than later when he was at an extreme of distress. Although this process clearly met a need, in my opinion, it was far from a satisfactory process.

3

DEFINING THE PROBLEM

*'A peaceful death must be acknowledged as a legitimate goal of
medicine, and as an integral part of the physician's responsibilities.'*
Dr Diane Meier (Editorial, *Annals of Internal Medicine*)[1]

Natural death—a declining phenomenon

In 2008, the idea of a natural death is becoming something of an
oxymoron. The occurrence of a natural death, uninfluenced by medical intervention, is increasingly uncommon, at least since the 1960s.[2]
Such deaths are very sudden, or occur during sleep. The commonest
causes of death are non-acute diseases such as cancer, cardio-respiratory
disease and neurological conditions (strokes and other chronic disorders).
Most people die in a way that is significantly influenced by medical
decisions regarding the manner and timing of their death. The
sociologist and philosopher Ivan Illich termed this invasiveness 'the
medicalisation of death'.[3] He claimed that modern medicine had
'brought the epoch of natural death to an end'.

One reputable study found that, for terminally ill cancer patients,
'more than 90% of patients required medical management for a major

symptom issue in the final week of life'.[4] Another large government-funded study found 'severe symptoms in the last three days of life in patients with heart failure; 65% were breathless and 42% had severe pain'.[5] In intensive care units, '74% of patients had some form of treatment withheld or withdrawn before death'.[6] New Zealand experts, writing about 'The Last 48 Hours of Life', found that 'most dying patients are on an opioid (morphine)' and yet 'of our patients, 51% suffered pain in the last 48 hours'.[7] Respiratory distress is particularly common in cardio-respiratory failure and also in terminal cancer. Declan Walsh from the prestigious Cleveland Clinic stated that 'it is unacceptable to allow patients to die with unrelieved respiratory distress—drug doses should be increased as required for this purpose, even at the risk of hastening death from central nervous system depression'.[8] Professor Erich Loewy confirmed this reality, stating that 'most patients are, in fact, sedated and given analgesics at the end of life'.[9] In summary, most deaths are medically managed, because of the over-riding and universally accepted necessity to relieve suffering.

It is quite clear that the suffering of some people will be relieved only by their death, or by being rendered unconscious by drugs until they die. Thus it is common to hear the comment from treating staff and relatives alike, when death finally occurs, 'I'm glad that's over' or 'What a merciful release'. It is also quite clear that a peaceful death cannot usually be achieved without significant medical intervention that has the potential to hasten death. Decisions that shorten life abound in medicine today, and are based on either the futility of further treatment or the necessity to relieve profound suffering. Such shortening of life is usually only a matter of hours, but may sometimes be days, even weeks and, very rarely, years. But who makes these decisions; who makes these choices?

The rise of patient autonomy
As managed death has developed, so too has a remarkable change in medical attitudes to patient autonomy. With the rise of human rights

movements, there came a challenge to the patronising attitudes of the medical profession. Feminism played a significant role, the majority of nurses being women. Citizens demanded more information and the courts upheld their right to be fully informed. They also wanted to be involved in decisions about treatment, and whether they would have any treatment at all. By 2000 the principle of autonomy had become the dominant ethic of health care in North America and Western Europe,[10] and it is true of Australia. Thus, in many jurisdictions the long-established, but little-used, common law right to refuse treatment was confirmed in statute law, even if such refusal of treatment would lead to a hastened death. In Victoria this took the form of the *Medical Treatment Act* (1988). This confirmation of the patient's autonomy arose directly from a Parliamentary Committee of Inquiry into Dying with Dignity. This Act also stated in its preamble that the Parliament recognised that it was desirable 'to ensure that dying patients receive maximum relief from pain and suffering'. It was this Act that established many of the guidelines for my practice. All the other states in Australia except New South Wales have developed similar legislation.

The language of a 'peaceful death'

For centuries, it has been medicine's aim to try to achieve a 'peaceful death', as Diane Meier calls it (see p. 19), or, as others might put it, a 'good death'. A 'good death' is the translation of the Greek word *euthanasia* (or perhaps to be more realistic, 'the least worst death', as the American philosopher Margaret Pabst Battin put it),[11] and this simple expression is clearly a desirable aim. But does a 'peaceful death' refer only to the moment of death, perhaps the last hour or so, or to the whole process that leads towards it? Most people are prepared to accept some pain and discomfort, but not the grosser forms of suffering that affect about 5 per cent of deaths.

Over the past forty years, there has been a vigorous debate as to how that 'good death' was to be achieved. This debate had been given real substance by medical practice in the Netherlands. There, in the 1960s and 1970s, hastening of death was practised covertly, often by anaesthetists. As a result, an anaesthetic method of an injected sedative (for deep sleep) and muscle relaxant (to stop breathing) became the usual practice. In 1973, the Dutch doctor mentioned earlier was charged with murder after she ended the life of her frail, elderly, suffering mother. She was found guilty, but not punished.[12] This led to intense debate, and ultimately the development of a set of medical practice guidelines. Provided these guidelines were followed and the assistance in death was reported, doctors assisting death by a lethal injection or, less commonly, by physician-assisted suicide (where the individual swallows lethal prescription medication) were not prosecuted. It is the practice of a lethal injection to relieve unbearable suffering that has virtually become synonymous with the modern use of the term euthanasia. Euthanasia is voluntary when the doctor acts in response to a request by the suffering person, and is extremely unlikely to be other than voluntary when that person actively ends their own life (as by the oral self-administration of a fatal dose).

The Remmelink Inquiry
The definition of euthanasia and its shortcomings

Voluntary euthanasia by lethal injection had been practised in the Netherlands without prosecution for some years. Provided the doctor followed the guidelines formulated by the Royal Dutch Medical Association in conjunction with government authorities he or she would not be prosecuted. The guidelines stipulated that deliberately hastened deaths must be reported to the Dutch equivalent of the Australian coroner. In 1985, the Dutch government, concerned about a suspected low level of reporting of voluntary euthanasia deaths, established the Remmelink Inquiry to obtain factual information about medical decisions at the end of life. The results of this official survey were published in 1991 in *The Lancet*, a prestigious British medical journal.[13] Its principal focus was on the question of euthanasia as described above (that is, by lethal injection), but it was also concerned to collect information about all other medical decisions affecting the end of life. These also included physician-assisted suicide (self-administered prescribed drugs), non-treatment decisions that shortened life, alleviation of pain with high doses of medication with at least the partial intention of hastening death, and also the use of high doses of medication that would have the probable (foreseeable) effect of shortening the patient's life—all, in fact, instances of medically influenced dying. Because the study was attempting to distinguish between the different kinds of hastened death that might occur, it had to devise a way of clearly and precisely separating these events that, from the clinician's point of view, may commonly overlap. As Dr FG Miller states, 'The intentions of clinicians may be multiple and ambiguous, and the causal contribution of escalating doses of morphine to the timing of terminally ill patients' deaths may be difficult to discern. Therefore there exists a grey zone between standard palliative care and active euthanasia'.[14] Since the study aimed to examine a range of 'medical decisions at the end of life' (MDELs), it needed to eliminate this 'grey zone' and therefore adopted the following definition for voluntary euthanasia: 'The prescription, supply or administration of drugs with the explicit intention of shortening life at the patient's request'.

This definition obviously includes voluntary euthanasia both by direct lethal injection administered by the doctor and by physician-assisted suicide (where the doctor prescribes the medication with the intention that the patient is free to ingest or personally administer it). The Remmelink definition rolls both these actions together, although there are significant differences between them. The definition focuses entirely on the intention of the doctor without any reference to the context of the action. This description was designed for the purposes of the empirical research but seemed to me to be inadequate as a clear definition of euthanasia. It was specifically used for the purpose of this study to distinguish these actions from others that, whilst differing in kind, nevertheless had essentially the same outcome and, at least partially, the same intention. While this definition was very useful for empirical research, it has skewed the debate ever since. This bald description can be paraphrased readily as indicating that voluntary euthanasia is simply the deliberate intention to kill, and has been so used in this way by opponents of voluntary euthanasia. This descriptor was intended to relate to people who were either terminally or hopelessly ill and who had great suffering, but it did not say so specifically. In the Dutch context, it was taken for granted.

Taking the Remmelink definition at face value, a doctor who supplies or administers drugs to a perfectly healthy young person with the intention of shortening their life, at their request, has committed euthanasia; or indeed, to any person, at any stage of life, regardless of the circumstances. This is simplistic and not, of course, what happens in the Netherlands. It is not what any serious advocate of voluntary euthanasia argues for, yet some opponents of voluntary euthanasia constantly state that this would be the outcome if legislation for voluntary euthanasia or physician-assisted suicide were passed. More importantly, the Remmelink definition describes an intention (which is subjective) instead of an action or effect (which is quantifiable).

Thus the Remmelink definition creates problems, first because it is entirely devoid of context (the presence of suffering and terminal illness), second because it defines by way of intention rather than effect, and, third, the intention is defined as to shorten life. It ignores what is, in my opinion, the primary intention of the doctor, namely to relieve suffering, or alternatively provide maximal palliation. For my own part, I see such actions as intended to palliate patients' intolerable suffering, while clearly hastening death (rapidly in the case of an injection, or more slowly if medication is ingested). In the latter case, it could even be argued that the doctor's intention is to give patients control over the end of their own life, whereas it is the patients' intention to end their own life.

There are, in fact, many definitions of euthanasia (and physician-assisted suicide). The World Medical Association defined it as 'the act of deliberately ending the life of a patient at the patient's own request';[15] the British House of Lords said it was 'a deliberate intervention undertaken with the express intention of ending a life to relieve intractable suffering';[16] the Catholic Church (Evangelium Vitae) said it was 'an action or omission which of itself and by intention causes death, with the purpose of eliminating all suffering'.[17] Ezekiel Emanuel, an American bioethicist, defined it as 'intentionally administering medications or other interventions to cause the patient's death at the patient's explicit request and with full informed consent'. All these, and other, definitions emphasise the intention of the doctor in 'ending life' or 'causing death', whilst others use language such as 'shortening life' or 'hastening death'. Some include the request of the person, and some include the relief of suffering, but none covers all aspects of this complex issue. It is noteworthy that the definition used by various Dutch bodies, but particularly the Royal Dutch Medical Association, changed frequently as greater understanding of the issues became clear through analysis of practice.

A doctor's intention in end-of-life decisions may be complex, ambiguous, multifactorial and uncertain, and an inadequate basis for legal definition. The ultimate Netherlands legislation of 2002 to legalise physician-assisted dying simply indicates that it is speaking of 'a doctor who terminates life on request' (this seems to ignore the possibility of the person terminating his or her own life, and highlights the Dutch emphasis, unfortunate to my mind, on lethal injections). The context follows in the detail of the Act, where the word euthanasia is not actually used.

The importance of context

Euthanasia in the Dutch sense does not occur simply because a doctor thinks it would be a good idea for a particular patient—it is not an abstract concept. It depends very much on context, and on context as judged by the suffering person. It occurs because that person, due to their circumstances, the context of their illness in relation to their life in all its facets, makes a decision to approach a doctor to ask for his or her help. The initiation of the dialogue that may lead to termination of life on request comes from the individual. It comes usually from their perception that their suffering is, or will become, intolerable and that their position is hopeless. It may also come from the possible misconception that they are doomed, that they will suffer intolerably in the future, and that they wish to avoid this presumed suffering at some time in the future. The doctor needs to gently challenge all these perceptions and possible misconceptions, and establish a rational basis for interaction. The doctor needs to look at the context in which the request is made and see if it can be changed, but if it cannot, then he must take the request seriously. Nevertheless, it should be the sufferer who initiates the dialogue.

People will not do this unless they are sorely tested by their circumstances. That person wants, above all, relief of suffering. The circumstances of two individuals are rarely the same, as each illness has a context beyond the mere physical component that affects decisions. Education, religion and beliefs, life experiences and social circumstances will all influence how people will react in a similar disease situation. There can be no simple rules as to whether or not a person might be making a rational request. This can be discovered only by detailed discussion. Similar influences will dictate how the individual doctor will react to a request.

The Remmelink definition describes the doctor's intention as being to shorten life (or hasten death, or deliberately kill). I profoundly disagree with this contention. I do not believe for one moment that a doctor contemplating euthanasia sets out in his or her mind to kill someone. Even though that may be the result, it is not the primary intention. The Remmelink definition is simplistic and ignores the complexity of medical intention in end-of-life decisions. What is the doctor's primary intention in providing a hastened death? Does he want to kill a human being? No. Does he want to kill a suffering human being? No, but he recognises that there may be no acceptable alternative. Does he want to relieve intolerable and unrelievable suffering because that is what that person requests? Clearly, yes. So his primary intention is to relieve suffering, while recognising that his action will hasten death, and will either kill that person or allow that person to kill himself. That is a clear consequence of his method, and is not denied, but it is very much a secondary intention, if it is that. There is a complexity in all end-of-life decisions between intention, motive, method and outcome. It is not what the doctor wants to do or desires to do but, in the circumstances, in order to act according to the expressed best interests of his patient, feels that it is necessary to do.

The starting point for the doctor's involvement is that he is confronted with a person who has profound suffering that is unrelievable except by either death or deep sleep maintained until death. Is there any difference except time? The intention of a doctor putting a patient into a deep coma to relieve intolerable suffering is no different from that of a doctor who either provides or administers medication that causes death quickly—in both instances the doctor's intention is to relieve intolerable suffering.

Dr Susan Chater analysed the attitudes of palliative care experts to terminal sedation (the deliberate sedation of a patient to unconsciousness, without the provision of fluids, that is maintained until they die). She found that 'the risk of undesirable outcome (shortening of life) is acceptable only because of the more compelling need to act to relieve suffering'.[18] It should be noted that the idea of death as an 'undesirable outcome' is the doctor's perception, but it may not be that of the patient. The Dutch, on the other hand, clearly recognise that terminal sedation (the intentional sedation to unconsciousness without provision of hydration) is a 'form of assistance in the dying process'. The fundamental difference between termination of life on request and aggressive palliative care by terminal sedation is that the doctor performing voluntary euthanasia acknowledges that his action *will* hasten death, perhaps almost instantaneously depending on method, whereas the palliative care doctor is at pains to declare that his treatment does not hasten death or, if reluctantly agreeing that it might have done so, argues that it was not his or her intention! But the fundamental intention of both doctors is the same, the intention to relieve intolerable suffering—the difference is the method they are using.

Dutch surgeon-oncologist Aycke Smook, who has had significant experience with voluntary euthanasia, defines euthanasia as 'an act performed by a physician on explicit request of a patient that involves injecting the lethal drug intravenously' and says 'the intent is a good death'.[19] Most important is the doctor's 'responsibility for the results of the intervention', whichever the type of intervention that shortens life.

The doctor's or the patient's intention?

The doctor who performs voluntary euthanasia or physician-assisted dying by whatever method has the primary intention of relieving his patient's suffering by maximal palliation. That person may well have the intention of ending his life as the only way to be relieved of that suffering. If you ask most people who request euthanasia if they want to die, they usually do not—their fundamental wish is for relief of suffering, but if that can occur only by way of death, then that is their intention. It is a mistake to focus on the intention of the doctor in this debate—he is secondary to the wishes and intentions of the person he is guiding in treatment. Cancer surgeon Charles McKhann echoes this view in his book *A Time to Die* when he says:

> End-of-life concerns should be focused on the patient rather than the physician or the law. Agony from advanced disease that is severe enough to make a person wish to have his life end is the same agony regardless of the mode of death, be it refusal of treatment, the double effect of drugs, suicide, assisted suicide, or euthanasia. The underlying reason that the patient wants earlier death is to end his suffering.[20]

It is empathy for the suffering of the individual and respect for the autonomy of that person's decision that leads the doctor to provide assistance. No suffering, no euthanasia; no request, no euthanasia. Both the request and the suffering belong to the sufferer—the doctor has no desire, nor any real intention, to hasten death, except in meeting the wishes and best interests of those for whom the doctor is caring.

Why is the intention of the doctor considered to be so important? Simply because the crimes of murder and assisting in suicide hang on the intention of the person who is involved in causing or hastening death. It is accepted legally that if a doctor hastens death while relieving suffering, then even though he could foresee that he might hasten death, he is not guilty if that was not his intention. Thus euthanasia is generally thought to be a crime because the commonly accepted definition (Remmelink) states that there is an explicit intention to shorten life, hasten death or, in extreme language, to kill.

While the person may decide to end his or her life in order to be relieved of his or her suffering, a further dimension of that decision is that death occurs in a dignified manner. Most dying people are capable of ending their lives in violent and undignified ways, and some do. No one should be forced to this despair for want of compassionate assistance.

My definition of voluntary euthanasia

The essential features of voluntary euthanasia, as I understand the term, are:

It is an act taken by an individual, or requested by that individual.
It is taken or requested by a rational, fully informed individual.
It is that individual's intention to be relieved of intolerable and otherwise unrelievable suffering.
It is an action that hastens death.
It is, for that individual, a dignified death.

The Remmelink definition includes only two of these features, and wrongly emphasises the intention of the doctor rather than that of the individual, and in my view is an inadequate and misleading definition. My definition for voluntary euthanasia is:

> An action taken by, or at the request of, a rational, fully informed individual, whose intention is to be relieved of intolerable and otherwise unrelievable suffering, that hastens death in a dignified manner.

Notably, this definition does not mention a doctor. He is not indispensable, although he is critically important to the individual's being fully informed and is the key to a dignified death.

It is with this meaning that I use this term in this book, qualifying the term as necessary to the method of voluntary euthanasia involved. This definition is a statement of principles. It is person-centred, recognising the centrality of the individual in medical decisions, and gives the individual responsibility for the decision. That person may also take the responsibility for the action (physician-assisted suicide) or negotiate with the doctor to provide a direct lethal injection if circumstances dictate this as the best or only option. Physician-assisted dying may involve a withdrawal or non-initiation of treatment, if it is associated with sedation that hastens death while relieving accompanying suffering, if that is the person's wish. It may even include deliberate sedation until death if the person felt that such a process had dignity.

Such a concept could be likened to the branches of a tree, all parts of a whole. The long-established method of increasing doses of morphine could be likened to the old gnarled trunk. Withholding of treatment is an old branch, while withdrawal of treatment has grown from it. Terminal sedation is a newer branch, but is now secure and established. Physician-assisted dying by injection or self-administration are also new branches, not yet strong enough to be accepted as secure and certain, but parts of that same tree nevertheless.

Euthanasia has become a maligned and abused word in modern times, a far cry from its original meaning of 'a good death'. This is largely because it lacks precise definition and means different things to different people. A 'good death' can be achieved in a variety of ways—that is, the method—but the principle is the same in all cases.

It is the relief of suffering by a palliative means that respects the wishes of the patient. It is a profoundly ethical medical principle and, as Diane Meier says, an integral medical responsibility or duty. Because of the influences of history and religion, we have reached an impasse where some ways of delivering a 'good death' are accepted and legal, while others are considered by some to be illegal and unacceptable. Unfortunately, these illegal methods are the methods that are most dignified and most acceptable to many people in the community, as polls of public opinion have persistently shown.[21]

Further confusion over terminology

To add to the confusion about terminology, some writers, particularly in America, have shown a tendency to conflate voluntary euthanasia by lethal injection and voluntary euthanasia by self-administered oral medication under the blanket heading of 'physician-assisted suicide'. They regard the request for assistance to die and the subsequent death by lethal injection as a form of suicide, in that it is a deliberate ending of one's own life. This argument has some substance where the person requesting assistance uses a computerised injection technique, allowing that person to control totally the delivery of the lethal medication (as was the case with Philip Nitschke's patients in the Northern Territory of Australia). However, there are significant practical and ethical differences between these approaches. The use of the term physician-assisted suicide in this way is confusing, and I do not use it in this sense in this book. For me, the term specifically means a death by self-administered oral medication (or very rarely via a stomach tube if oral access is impossible) with the physician assisting by advice and prescription.

'Suicide' in English means the deliberate taking of one's own life. It has come to be associated with mental illness, irrationality, shame and, in the minds of some, sin. As a result it carries an enormous negative stigma. Unfortunately, there is no easy way to differentiate the suicide of a person who (perhaps from transient psychological distress) irrationally ends their life from one with intolerable and unrelievable suffering who, calmly and after due consideration, rationally does so. An irrational, or ill-considered, suicide is one undertaken in the confused and mistaken belief that circumstances are irrevocably dismal and improvement impossible, when, in fact, that is objectively not so to an impartial and experienced observer. A rational suicide, on the other hand, is undertaken after a careful assessment of the circumstances, concluding that they are not going to get better; in fact, they will only get worse, no matter what is done. Many would argue that the term 'suicide' is not appropriate to use in the latter circumstance, but there is no alternative, except to qualify it as a 'rational suicide' or to describe it in broader terms as 'physician-assisted dying by self-administration'.

Because all of the above methods of euthanasia are essentially medical methods of hastening death, they are all examples of 'physician-assisted dying'. Where such physician-assisted dying is associated with a patient's intention to be relieved of suffering and request for a hastened but dignified death, it becomes an alternative expression for voluntary euthanasia, but lacks the pejorative and confused connotations of that term. Unfortunately, so much of the confusion about voluntary euthanasia revolves around differing views about what it actually is—different perceptions and ways of interpreting and understanding actions, and differing meanings placed on words. This is well illustrated by the statement of Dr John Zalcberg, a Melbourne palliative care physician, who said:

> it is true that when people are within days or weeks of the ends
> of their lives, the introduction of morphine can lead to an alter-
> ation of their conscious state. We accept this as an inevitable effect
> of treating pain at the end of people's lives, their length of life
> being determined by their disease. If the pain is well controlled
> the dose of morphine is kept constant. We aim to have patients
> awake and alert, but if the patient is not awake at the time their
> pain is controlled, we accept that as an inevitable consequence

... Is that euthanasia? I think some doctors would say it is. I believe it is symptom control. But if it is euthanasia then, yes, we practice euthanasia.[22]

This is effectively an admission that there is no practical distinction between palliative care and euthanasia, not one that words can clearly differentiate. Euthanasia, as I define it, could be considered the most effective form of palliation of intolerable and unrelievable suffering, from the suffering individual's point of view.

A result of this confusion

On 4 March 2003, David Armstrong (former editor-in-chief of *The Australian*) related, in his paper, the heart-rending story of his wife's death from motor neurone disease (MND; a disease to which I will refer often in this book). His story illustrates the all too frequent lack of communication between doctor and patient when that person is dying. As a result, there exists a fundamental ignorance about physician-assisted dying in any form. He said, 'Her life expectancy was much shorter than the usual three or so years from diagnosis. But the doctor didn't tell us that'. A little later:

> One of the doctors warned me [not his wife] that she would soon suffer great distress. 'You won't want to see it, and you certainly won't want the girls to watch their mum going through it. When that time comes, call me and we'll put her into hospital and make her comfortable'. I didn't know what it meant. I thought it may mean euthanasia but I also thought that couldn't be right. So I didn't know what to expect and I wasn't going to ask. I was too afraid to do so.

Armstrong was left with the terminal care of his wife at home (their choice) with the assistance of nurses, and possibly an overview by palliative care, and a doctor's advice by phone! The last few days, as described by Armstrong, were appalling. His wife became 'highly distressed physically and emotionally as she struggled to breathe. A nurse told me Deb should be in hospital. I couldn't even contemplate it. I didn't know what *they would do*'. His wife was asking to be assisted to die at home—she had known of gay friends who had achieved this, but she was denied. There was no doctor in sight and it was almost too late for such a dialogue. Armstrong had to manage his own wife's death, not quite alone, but with only 'nod nod, wink wink' advice from the medical profession. Morphine was prescribed to make Deb 'comfortable', 'and it did, after a fashion'. 'The morphine was not enough to keep her under, so the periods of struggle kept returning.' In the end, Armstrong requested an additional dose of morphine and his wife died.

The distraught husband was now haunted by the question, 'Did we kill Deb?' Although reassured by friends, relations and nurses, 'that still didn't stop the nightmares'. This unfortunate family had been caught up in dying 2003-palliative style, in which discussion of dying was taboo, communication was lacking and honesty was a victim to hypocrisy. Inadequate relief of suffering was the outcome. Armstrong, an intelligent man, was swamped by a lack of communication and assistance, by a fog of moral confusion, and engulfed by guilt and nightmares, and yet he could still say, 'I'm sure that dying peacefully with friends and family around her was better than being deliberately helped from this world. It was certainly better for me—and for our children. I'm sure it was better for Deb too'.

How would he know? It might be a comforting thought to rationalise what actually happened. But how could he possibly know of an alternative of which he had no experience? How much does any Australian really know about the context of voluntary euthanasia? The administration of morphine had provided a degree of necessary palliation, but nevertheless there had been heart-rending unrelieved suffering for about three days. How much better might her palliation have been if voluntary euthanasia were seen as what it really is—not deliberate killing, but the most effective means of palliation, if that is the person's choice.

4

A NAÏVE DEATH

'My God, my God, why hast thou forsaken me?'
Jesus Christ (St Mark, 15:34)

'I cannot and will not recant, for it is neither wise nor salutary to act against one's conscience.'
Martin Luther (18 April 1521, *Diet of Worms*)

Len was sixty-five when he came to my out-patient clinic at the Austin Hospital in Melbourne in the mid-1970s, complaining of some months of intermittent bleeding when urinating, which he had unfortunately neglected. He also needed to urinate frequently and with embarrassing urgency. This combination of symptoms left me very concerned that he might be suffering from a bladder cancer infiltrating deeply into the bladder wall, and so it proved to be. Investigation confirmed that his cancer was very aggressive and was not curable by surgery. He was advised to have radiation therapy with the rather forlorn hope of cure, but the greater hope that this treatment would alleviate his symptoms.

This treatment was not effective as, on follow-up examination, cancer persisted in his bladder and he returned at regular intervals to the hospital with increasing symptoms of bleeding, and frequency and urgency of urination with significant pain and incontinence. His bleeding often resulted in clots forming in his bladder, which blocked his flow of urine, causing great pain. His bladder had undergone significant contraction as a result of the radiation therapy, so that his pain on becoming obstructed was extreme.

Len underwent a number of telescopic examinations of his bladder, in an attempt to control his cancer and stop his bleeding, which were of limited value. He required a series of blood transfusions to correct the anaemia caused by his persistent bleeding. Len's general health was steadily deteriorating, with lethargy and weight loss, due to the progressive ravages of the cancer.

Len was widowed and lived alone. Fortunately, he had the assistance of a loving daughter who visited him regularly and helped him manage at home, but Len's life was becoming a misery. I remember picking up his file one morning in the out-patient department with some trepidation. I realised that a most difficult consultation was now before me because Len's illness was reaching a very difficult phase. He was approaching death and medicine's ability to palliate him was severely limited. Any treatment that would prolong his life would inevitably prolong his suffering.

Len entered my consulting room looking as pale as chalk. He told me that he had been bleeding persistently for some time and was having difficulty with the passage of clots from his bladder. He needed to urinate every fifteen minutes with such a great sense of urgency that he often wet himself. The pain on attempting to urinate was often excruciating. It was episodic in nature and not at a consistent level, making it particularly difficult to palliate with oral medication.

Such diabolical suffering was the reason that generations of surgeons had whispered the aphorism, 'Please God, do not take me through my bladder'. This plea had originated from the agonies of the era of bladder stones, but is even more apposite to bladder cancer. It is personalised by the comment of John Arbuthnot, physician and wit from Queen Anne's time and the creator of 'John Bull'. Suffering grievously from a bladder stone, he wrote to his friend the novelist Jonathon Swift: 'A recovery is in my case and in my age impossible; the kindest wish of my friends is euthanasia'.

As I sat across the desk from Len, I felt a sense of enormous impotence—there was very little I could do that would significantly alter his level of physical and emotional suffering. I remember telling him that all I could do was once again bring him into hospital, place a catheter into his bladder to wash out any clots, give him a blood transfusion to restore his blood count, and perhaps perform a further telescopic examination of the bladder to try to stop the bleeding. Len's face on the other side of the desk was blank—he had been through this process on four previous occasions and he fully understood that this treatment would not only be very distressing, but be of little if any benefit. In both our minds, I am sure, it represented an exercise in futility that would lead to further inevitable suffering, and very soon at that.

Len looked me straight in the eye and said, 'Isn't there anything else you can do for me?' I will never forget Len's question as it is one of the most profound questions in medicine.

It jolted me to the core and reminds me now of the question asked by Jesus Christ, when on the cross, of his Father when he said, 'My God, my God, why hast thou forsaken me?' It is a question that comes from the depths of despair and the depths of intolerable suffering, and it surely cannot be met by a flippant answer.

Since the death of Betty in 1972, I had been thinking seriously about the correct medical response to unrelievable pain and intolerable suffering. Unfortunately, it is not uncommon for doctors to avoid this difficult discussion with their patient in front of them. It involves telling them that there is no further effective treatment and that they are dying. It is one of the hardest things a doctor ever has to do, but there are times when they must do it. They may be rather inclined to busy themselves in further futile investigations, experimental or otherwise debilitating and futile treatments, or handball the problem they are not prepared to address to another doctor, such as an oncologist or palliative care physician. Their unfortunate colleague is then expected to either produce a miracle or develop a rapport with a frightened and desperate patient late in the day. The patient is in danger of becoming a 'medical pawn', pushed hither and thither by his doctors in order to avoid the only question that matters.

Len had saved me from falling into that trap by his profound and abrupt question. Since Betty's death, I had come to the broad conclusion that if intolerable suffering was present, then that human being had a perfect right to ask for medication with the potential to end their life if that was the only way to end their suffering. It struck me that Len was in this position—but was he asking me that question? If he was, then I felt in conscience that I could not deny him.

There was a prolonged silence as I weighed up the meaning of his question. Was Len asking me for treatment that would relieve him of his suffering? If so, then the only treatment I could offer him was a quantity of sedatives with which he could go to sleep and not wake up, if he so chose. The out-patient department of a public hospital in 1976 was not a safe and private environment, and was not the ideal place to embark on a detailed and delicate conversation to explore his question. I had yet to learn the enormous importance of open dialogue between doctor and patient in this context.

I presumed that I understood Len's question and said, 'I can write you a prescription for some sleeping tablets—you can go home and take them and they may relieve your problem'. I will never forget the look of intense relief and simultaneous gratitude that suddenly illuminated Len's pallid face as his wish was granted. His reaction left me in no doubt that my interpretation of his question was correct.

To this point, however, I had not given the slightest consideration to how to implement a decision to assist somebody to die; I had thought about the problem from a philosophical point of view, but not from a practical point of view. I had no knowledge of what was an effective dose of medication that would help to palliate suffering by ending life. Now I was facing that decision with Len. I took Len's prescription book and wrote a prescription for the maximum allowable number of simple sleeping tablets. I advised him that if he took these he would go to sleep and probably not wake up.

How naïve was I? This commonly used sleeping tablet was hardly likely to hasten death and the quantity prescribed was hopelessly insufficient. I had reacted in a spontaneous fashion and in ignorance, driven by my compelling sense of necessity to help relieve Len's appalling suffering, and to help him to seek the peace of mind he yearned.

Confirmation of Len's extreme suffering came as he went straight home and took all the medication, and he did go to sleep. Two days later, his daughter called to see him and there was no response to her knock. She called the police who broke into the house and found Len deeply unconscious. Fortunately, he was readmitted to hospital under my care, and my colleagues were helpful in quietly acquiescing with my decision to simply keep him comfortable and to not prolong his life by treating his chest infection. I felt embarrassed when, on his admission to hospital, I realised how ineffectual and unfortunate my action had been. He remained mostly unconscious for a few days, though gradually recovered some consciousness before he died of respiratory complications one week after ingesting the tablets.

My action had assisted in hastening Len's death indirectly, because the consequence of his taking an 'overdose' of sedatives was the development of fatal pneumonia. My intention had been to allow Len to take control of his suffering, but I had not succeeded in giving Len the peace and control he desired, even though the sedatives had diminished his suffering. It was not, I'm sure, what Len had envisaged and it had certainly caused a great deal of distress to his daughter, with whom he had not discussed this matter. I realised that my action had been naïve in the extreme, and if I were to attempt to help other people making such requests in the future I would need to be more thoroughly prepared and communicate more effectively, and to encourage my patient to communicate with his family. Len missed the chance to say goodbye, and his daughter was deeply distressed. There was clearly no place for presumption, for not exploring the issues in depth. Acting by way of a 'wink and a nod', or with medications that were ineffective, was not acceptable and was courting disaster.

I thought that with Len's death and the signing of the death certificate the matter was ended. My confidence was shattered when, some weeks later, I received a phone call from a detective from the Criminal Investigation Branch who asked me why I had prescribed sedatives for Len. I took a very deep breath while trying to gather my thoughts. When I wrote Len's prescription, I had responded in a completely spontaneous manner out of empathy and an innate sense of wanting to help another human being who was in great suffering. This phone call brought me back to stark reality. I told the policeman that I had prescribed the medication because Len was having trouble sleeping. This was partly true but not in essence the real truth. The policeman accepted this explanation, with a stern warning to be careful in my prescribing habits, and I heard no more about the matter. However, his call impressed on me the fine line that a doctor runs when attempting to relieve suffering with treatment that has the potential to hasten death.

This sudden confrontation by the authorities made me fully aware that what I had done was potentially a very serious crime. The Victorian *Crimes Act* (Section 6B) states:

(2) Any person who—(a) incites any other person to commit suicide and that other person commits or attempts to commit suicide in consequence thereof; or

(b) aids or abets any other person in the commission of suicide or in an attempt to commit suicide—

shall be guilty of an indictable offence and liable to be imprisoned for a term of not more than fourteen years.

I realised at this point that I had commenced on a 'life of crime', and that if future patients like Len were to come to me for help, I would have no option, in all conscience, but to continue in this 'life of crime'. Betty had suffered excruciating pain and my relative had suffered excruciating breathing difficulty—very obvious physical suffering. Len had not only severe pain but also gross dysfunction of his bladder with uncontrollable incontinence, a subtle movement into the realm of loss of dignity. I was beginning to see in front of me the nature of suffering at the end of life. One thing was crystal clear—there are limits to each person's suffering. The words of Jesus Christ that head this chapter clearly confirm that even the Son of God sought relief from his intolerable suffering. Believers might think that perhaps God granted it.

5

A HOT POTATO

'As a palliative care professional, I oppose euthanasia as a personal choice, but I support its legislation. I will always try to talk you out of that choice. But if you can stand it no longer I would understand your wish to act and go. I would support your autonomy because you are a free citizen in a multicultural society, and not the plaything of clinical and religious institutions.'

Allan Kellehear, Professor of Palliative Care, La Trobe University

In early 1992, Professors Helga Kuhse and Peter Singer, from the Monash University Centre for Human Bioethics, published the results of a large survey of the attitudes of Victorian nurses to euthanasia (the Dutch definition).[1] It found that 55 per cent had been asked by a patient to hasten their death, and that 5 per cent of these had complied with a patient's direct request to explicitly end his or her life without having been asked by a doctor to do so. Seventy-five per cent indicated that they supported the introduction in Victoria of conditions regarding euthanasia similar to those in the Netherlands, and 65 per cent indicated that they would be willing to be involved in the provision of voluntary euthanasia if it were legal.

Since treating Len in 1976, I had been contemplating these matters seriously. As a result, I had come to the view that the appropriate medical response to valid and considered requests for assistance in dying was by way of the prescription of oral medication that would place the individual in control. This was in contrast to the Dutch solution of delivering a lethal injection. During that time I had experience of withdrawal of treatment and appropriate palliation, but I had not had any patients in my own practice who requested assistance in hastening death. In 1987, I had written a letter to *The Age* advocating a change to the law of this kind. Supporters of legislative reform noted this, and began to send me information. Subsequently, I received a few compelling requests from dying people who did not have a urological problem. I had published an article in the *Medical Journal of Australia* in February 1991[2] about Dr Jack Kevorkian (the American pathologist who had been charged with assisting suicide) in which I had spelt out my views on physician-assisted suicide as a means of physician-assisted dying, and I was becoming known as a doctor who would talk on these matters.

A journalist contacted me for comment on Kuhse and Singer's results. During the conversation, I mentioned that I had assisted three patients to die by provision of medication. I also discussed the death of Len in 1976. This revelation was entirely unpremeditated on my part. This was my first press interview on this subject and, stupidly, I did not realise that my comments could or would be reported. Once again, I was to behave in a very naïve manner in thinking that these admissions would not be fully exploited by the journalist.

I woke on Sunday, 8 March 1992, to read banner headlines on the front page of *The Sunday Age*—'I helped patients die: doctor'—and to a very busy phone. One call that I particularly remember was from an old friend of mine, a barrister now living in Queensland, who rang to warn me in the strongest terms not to say anything more on the subject lest I get into very serious trouble. It was kind of him, but by this stage I had given many interviews, and if I was in trouble, the die was already cast.

A fierce debate raged over the next fortnight in the Melbourne media, and beyond, but I was not contacted by anyone involved in the prosecution of the law. The barrister's dire warning was not fulfilled, and for the first time I began to feel that the authorities were not particularly interested in pursuing doctors who possibly broke the law while treating their terminal patients, provided no specific complaint was made.

Mark Ragg, a doctor and freelance journalist who specialised in writing on medical matters, wrote an excellent summary of this episode. *The Lancet* published the following article:

Debate over euthanasia has peaked in Australia in the past month because of two coincidental events.

A urologist in Victoria, Dr Rodney Syme, admitted publicly that on several occasions he had prescribed lethal doses of medication to terminally ill patients who he knew intended to take their own lives. He said that he supported euthanasia and was willing to go to court to defend the right to die an easy death. He was convinced that no jury would convict him, even though in Australia euthanasia is illegal.

In the days after Dr Syme's admission, several academics argued their points of view publicly. But the only authority giving a clear message was the Catholic Church, which said that it opposed euthanasia strongly. The office of the Victorian Attorney-General, the state's senior legal officer, declined to comment and said that it was a matter for the police. The police did not contact Mr Syme. Senior officials of the Australian Medical Association took several different positions which, if not conflicting, are confusing. They praised Dr Syme's bravery in making the issue public and sympathized with his actions. Yet they emphasized that they did not condone his actions, which were illegal ...

At the same time, the Australian Government's Office of Film and Literature Classification decided to ban the import of *Final Exit*, a practical guide to suicide written by Derek Humphry, who is an active supporter of euthanasia …

Although unrelated, the two events reveal conflicting attitudes among Australian governments and institutions. They also reveal how desperately most governments and institutions want to avoid having to confront the legal position of euthanasia … Euthanasia is no longer automatically condemned, but neither is it publicly supported. The ambivalence of governments and legal and health authorities suggests that public debate is required to allow all the issues to be clarified. The difficulty is that many are prepared to call for more debate on the issue, but few are prepared to air their views.[3]

So the matter died in the media, but not with respect to my medical practice. That exposure and admission made me a target for referrals from other doctors, but more particularly for phone calls and letters from an increasing number of patients with very persuasive stories to tell. The next sixteen years became a roller-coaster ride that thoroughly tested my conscience. It involved sixteen years of helping patients to die in order to relieve their suffering, potentially breaking the law and confronting authority in the process.

6

CROSSING THE LINE

'The only purpose for which power can be rightfully exercised over any member of a civilized community, against his will, is to prevent harm to others. His own good, either physical or moral, is not sufficient warrant.'
John Stuart Mill (1806–1873), *On Liberty*

'If I lose my honour, I lose myself.'
Mark Antony (*Antony and Cleopatra*, William Shakespeare)

In March 1991, I read an article in the *New England Journal of Medicine* that moved me to tears and significantly affected my practice of medicine. It was by Timothy Quill, an American physician and palliative care specialist, who has written extensively on dying with dignity, but was unknown to me at the time. The article was entitled 'Death with dignity—a case of individualized decision making', and it described his involvement with his patient 'Diane', who was suffering from a highly malignant leukaemia. Rather than undergo aggressive chemotherapy and a bone marrow transplant with only a 25 per cent chance of 'cure', she elected to be given 'comfort care' (simple treatment to alleviate symptoms) and to spend her remaining time productively with her family and friends.

Quill, a lifelong advocate of patient autonomy, agreed with her decision after ensuring she was fully informed to make such an important decision. What happened next is best described in Quill's own words:

> Just as I was adjusting to her decision, she opened up another area that would stretch me profoundly. It was extraordinarily important to Diane to maintain control of herself and her own dignity during the time remaining to her. When this was no longer possible, she clearly wanted to die. As a former director of a hospice program, I know how to use pain medicines to keep patients comfortable and to lessen suffering. I explained the philosophy of comfort care, which I strongly believe in. Although Diane understood and appreciated this, she had known of people lingering in what is called relative comfort, and she wanted no part of it. When the time came, she wanted to take her life in the least painful way possible. Knowing of her desire for independence and her decision to stay in control, I thought this request made perfect sense. I acknowledged and explored this wish but also thought that it was out of the realm of currently accepted medical practice and that it was more than I could offer or promise. In our discussion, it became clear that preoccupation with her fear of a lingering death would interfere with Diane's getting the most out of the time she had left until she found a safe way to ensure her death. I feared the effects of a violent death on her family, the consequences of an ineffective suicide that would leave her lingering in precisely the state she dreaded so much, and the possibility that a family member would be forced to assist her, with all the legal and personal repercussions that would follow. She discussed this at length with her family. They believed that they should respect her choice. With this in mind, I told Diane that information was available from the Hemlock Society that might be helpful to her.

A week later she phoned me with a request for barbiturates for sleep. Since I knew that this was an essential ingredient in a Hemlock Society suicide, I asked her to come to the office to talk things over. She was more than willing to protect me by participating in a superficial conversation about her insomnia, but it was important to me to know how she planned to use the drugs and to be sure that she was not in despair or overwhelmed in a way that might color her judgment. In our discussion, it was apparent that she was having trouble sleeping, but it was evident that the security of having enough barbiturates available to commit suicide when and if the time came would leave her secure enough to live fully and concentrate on the present. It was clear that she was not despondent and that in fact she was making deep, personal connections with her family and close friends. I made sure that she knew how to use the barbiturates for sleep, and also that she knew the amount needed to commit suicide. We agreed to meet regularly, and she promised to meet with me before taking her life, to ensure that all other avenues had been exhausted. I wrote the prescription with an uneasy feeling about the boundaries I was exploring—spiritual, legal, professional, and personal. Yet I also felt strongly that I was setting her free to get the most out of the time she had left, and to maintain dignity and control on her own terms until her death.[1]

These two paragraphs crystallised my thoughts and expressed as clearly as possible the philosophy I had been groping towards. No wonder George Annas, a noted American medico-legal analyst, said after reading this article, 'I want this guy as my doctor'. Paradoxically, Annas opposes the legalisation of physician-assisted dying. After a few fruitful weeks, Diane took her life, alone, to protect her family. Quill's story continues:

Diane taught me about the range of help I can provide if I know people well and if I allow them to say what they really want. She taught me about life, death, and honesty and about taking charge and facing tragedy squarely when it strikes. She taught me that I can take small risks for people that I really know and care about. Although I did not assist her suicide directly, I helped indirectly to make it possible, successful and relatively painless. Although I know we have measures to help control pain and lessen suffering, to think that people do not suffer in the process of dying is an illusion. Prolonged dying can occasionally be peaceful, but more often the role of the physician and family is limited to lessening but not eliminating severe suffering.

I wonder how many families and physicians secretly help patients over the edge into death in the face of severe suffering. I wonder how many severely ill or dying patients secretly take their lives, dying alone in despair. I wonder whether the image of Diane's final aloneness will persist in the minds of her family, or if they will remember more the intense, meaningful months they had together before she died. I wonder whether Diane struggled in that last hour, and whether the Hemlock Society's way of death by suicide is the most benign. I wonder why Diane, who gave so much to so many of us, had to be alone for the last hour of her life.[2]

Seventeen years on, this writing still touches me, both in the heart and in the mind, in a profound way. Quill opened my mind to another level of medical practice and remains a hero in a world where heroes are scarce. When 'Diane's' identity was subsequently revealed, Quill was arraigned before a Grand Jury, a harrowing experience, but it was found that he had no case to answer. It was not considered that he had assisted in Diane's suicide! So many questions, and sixteen years on, still no answers.

As a result of the March 1992 publicity in *The Age*, I was contacted in January 1993 by a lady whose mother was suffering from advanced multiple sclerosis. Alice had extreme difficulty in speaking and writing. Her daughter asked if I would visit her at her home to talk about physician-assisted dying. The little information she gave me was compelling.

When I had helped Len it had been the result of an impulsive, naïve reaction, carried out on the spur of the moment, without any prior consideration. There was no direct request and no specific advice, just a vague understanding. This was different. This was an explicit request and would require detailed consideration of all the aspects of the matter, and it was extremely likely that the issue would become even more demanding after I met her, and as the facts emerged. While I could always say no at any time, I knew in my mind and heart that, once involved, I would find it very difficult in conscience to withdraw. It would be cruel to engage Alice in a dialogue if I was not prepared to follow through. This was a critical decision time for me—did I have the courage to do what I believed was right when it meant potentially coming into serious conflict with the law?

My conscience won out and I agreed to see her. I drove to her home on a Saturday morning, found the house and drove on, parking some distance away. I did not want anyone to remember my car parked outside her house for some time. Alice was in her fifties. She had suffered from multiple sclerosis for some years, and she was now in an advanced stage. Her husband was nearly twenty years older and had looked after her in their home in a most devoted fashion, with the help of their daughter. Alice was totally paralysed in both legs and one arm, and the other arm was becoming progressively useless. She was legally blind, due to the disease. She had no control of her bladder and bowel, and was permanently catheterised. She was essentially bed-bound, as contractures of the limbs made it difficult to sit in a wheelchair, and these deformed joints caused her pain. When I met her and her family, she was lying on a padded trolley. Her voice was affected by the disease and tired easily, so that she had difficulty with communication. She was totally dependent, and it was only through the dedication of her husband and daughter, and a lot of external assistance, that she was able to remain at home. This was important to her, but could not continue indefinitely, as her older husband was finding it increasingly difficult to cope, and she was faced with the prospect of permanent nursing home placement.

Multiple sclerosis is a disease of unknown cause, which has an inexorable course of progressive muscular paralysis, sometimes with temporary remissions, but in addition to paralysis of muscles can affect vision and bladder function in a disastrous way. There is no cure. Treatment is simply the attempt to minimise its ravages with good physical and nursing care. In its later stages it may be one of the classic hopeless illnesses. This is an illness without cure, which runs a prolonged course, sometimes in a stepwise manner until a sudden death, or progressively downhill to an inevitably degrading death, and with no means to relieve the associated physical, psychological and existential suffering.

Alice told me how, two years before, she had taken a large amount of heroin tablets with the intention of ending her life. She had no medical advice about this, but did become unconscious. However, some hours later, she had not died. Her husband panicked and called a doctor. A young locum doctor from an emergency service, who did not know her, responded. He agreed to the family's request that she not be resuscitated, but that she be transferred to the local public hospital to ensure adequate comfort care. Her husband was her legally appointed agent under the Victorian *Medical Treatment Act*, which gave him the power to refuse any medical treatment other than palliative care. He requested that she not be resuscitated, but despite this, the emergency doctors insisted on treatment. After further protest by her husband, the Public Advocate was called to interview her, and although her husband believed she was still under the influence of drugs and could not subsequently remember the interview, permission was given by the Public Advocate for the performance of an operation (tracheostomy— to aid breathing) and the administration of antibiotics. Thus she survived and spent three weeks in hospital, her legacy of the visit being a scar on her throat (as well as her psyche), a much weakened voice and a deep fear of failing in any future attempt to end her life.

I asked her if she had any regrets about the previous failed suicide attempt, or was she glad that it had failed. She clearly regretted her resuscitation, and as a result of that experience was fearful of making another attempt. She was also fearful of implicating her family in possible criminal charges, as her disability was rapidly taking the choice of helping herself out of reach. It was clear to me that her family must have rendered some assistance in her failed suicide attempt and had already run a significant risk in trying to help her. She did not want to expose them to further risk.

The courts of all the states of Australia have been demeaned by a series of prosecutions over the past fifteen years for murder, attempted murder, assisted suicide and manslaughter by loving relatives ('mercy killings'), who, through reasons of love and compassion, have hastened, or attempted to hasten, the deaths of their close relatives to end their suffering. In virtually every case, despite the charge being of a very serious nature, the judge imposed an insignificant or suspended penalty. Some recent judicial comments are worth noting. In 2003, Justice Coldrey of the Victorian Supreme Court stated, in sentencing a man pleading guilty to assisting his wife's suicide when she was suffering from terminal cancer, that the deceased had been a very private person 'who was very concerned about being in control of her own destiny' and 'was quite rational on the morning she died'. He handed down a suspended sentence. In 2004, Justice Peter Underwood of the Tasmanian Supreme Court, in another case of assisted suicide, inflicted no penalty on a son who helped his frail, dependent 88-year-old mother to end her life. He said, 'Curiously, it might be said that those who wish to end their life, but are physically unable to do so, are discriminated against by reason of their disability'. In 2005, Newcastle magistrate Alan Railton had to sentence an elderly man who had smothered his wife of forty-three years, whom he had nursed for sixteen years with multiple sclerosis that had progressed to quadriplegia. Terrified of ending in a nursing home, she had asked him to end her life. Railton handed down a suspended sentence, which was not surprising, but in a unique and significant act, he allowed the man to walk directly from the court with his barrister and friends rather than the normal practice of returning the sentenced person to the cells before release. Clearly Railton did not see him as a criminal or his action as a crime. The Australian judiciary has been sending a persistent signal to our parliaments on the issue of 'mercy killing', but our politicians have been deaf to this signal.

I could not deny that Alice had serious impairment of her quality of life, and that she had a permanent untreatable and hopeless illness. Her circumstances created utterly intolerable suffering as far as she was concerned. Even if I had any doubt of this, expert advice was quite clear—'Clinicians would do well to remember that when their assessment of quality of life is at odds with that of the patient, it is the patient who should have the final word.'[3] She knew her care was an enormous burden to her husband and family, and she wanted her husband to have some quality to his remaining life. Although he had shouldered this burden willingly and stoically, this did not alter the fact that, for her, it was a very real burden that she no longer wanted to impose. Two years ago, her situation had been desperate enough for her to attempt suicide, and now she was in an even worse situation. She was rapidly losing the function of her right hand and thus the ability to help herself. I empathised with her completely, and resolved to try to help her.

But how could this be achieved? I was not her treating doctor, and as a urologist could have no reasonable clinical connection to her except that she had a chronic urinary infection due to her catheter. I was not in a position to prescribe drugs with likely fatal consequences without the probability of awkward questions if she used them to take her life. Two possibilities existed—she might have effective drugs in her possession or she might get them from her general practitioner. He was an excellent doctor who gave her very good care, but was not cooperative with her wish to die and had told her that she must learn to adapt to the situation! No luck there. Her own drugs were many and varied—anti-spasmodics, simple sedatives, antidepressants and simple analgesics—but nothing that, on its own, would end her life reliably with both security and dignity. Above all else, this woman needed certainty that what she attempted would be successful. All I could do at this stage was empathise with her dilemma, and suggest that she try to find another local doctor who might be more sympathetic. I explained in detail how the law should operate (it had not appeared to do so two years before) and gave her my categorical assurance that if she made another suicide attempt, I would be prepared to admit her to hospital under my care and ensure that her refusal of treatment was honoured. I explained how dangerous it would be for me to prescribe drugs for her, but promised to do some research to find a way with her medications to achieve what she wanted, an end to her suffering.

One week later, I received this typed letter from her.

Thank you very much for your kind visit to my house approx. a week ago.

I am most anxious to be in a more definite position to have some control and to have means to exercise my decision by myself, while I still can.

I realise that I can not be helped by anybody directly, but I still lack the certain knowledge as to what would help me, and what is available.

Perhaps you would know indirectly of a person, that can help me with a precise information, and where I can get the necessary materials.

I am literally trapped in a situation, where my life would be unbearable if my absolutely total disabilities to which I am now very close, were to disable my weak right hand and my mind to a no hope of rescue situation, for the rest of my intolerable life.

My husband and family have been wonderful to me, but my husband is nearing seventy and I think he will soon not be able to look after me, and I could not tolerate total helplessness in a nursing home.

Her spidery, anguished and nearly illegible signature followed. Her dilemma could not have been more starkly expressed. Clearly I had been ambivalent in my advice to her, and had not given her much confidence that I would help her. I was still struggling with my own thoughts of whether to take a quite deliberate decision to break the law in order to help her in an action that I felt was completely justified. I was hoping that she could find someone else to help her, such as another local general practitioner, to get me off the hook. This hope was dashed when her husband rang to tell me that he could not find another GP who would do house calls, which were essential, let alone begin a discussion about the sensitive and dangerous subject of assisting suicide. I was, as I originally suspected, trapped. I simply could not walk away from Alice and leave her to even worse suffering than she already had. The simple fact was that her suffering would be ended only by her death.

Her letter indicated not only the desire to make her own decision but the reasons for this. She expressed the need to have control, which, if obtained, will allow many people to carry on in desperate circumstances. Clearly, her suffering had an enormous psychological element as she envisaged even greater entrapment in the very near future. The existential issues of total dependence and permanent incarceration in a nursing home were dominant.

Seale and Addington-Hall found dependency important in causing the feeling that an earlier death would have been better, and that it led to requests for euthanasia.[4] Loewy believes that 'what most patients fear most is powerlessness' and 'when all is said and done, powerlessness, social isolation and incapacitation are more feared than pain'.[5] Alice made little mention of her physical suffering, great though it was, revealing how suffering in the mind can outweigh all physical suffering. Her concern for her family was evident, as was her appreciation of their help. She was not acting out of any sense of duress.

I pondered how she could use the drugs that she had to end her life with security, but also with dignity. Her sedative was one that is rarely fatal even if taken in massive quantities (it was the one Len had taken), but she had enough to send her to sleep deeply for some days. She did have a quantity of antidepressants, a group of drugs that have been used successfully for suicide, but I could not find any reliable evidence about her particular drug or the quantities that might be needed. Above all, she needed something that would be totally reliable. She was taking paracetamol for pain, and I had seen vague references to its apparently quite common use in attempted suicide. I carried out a literature search in my hospital library and found a reference to 'acute liver necrosis following overdose of paracetamol'. This paper, published in 1966, was one of the first to draw attention to the fatal consequences of an overdose of paracetamol. A more recent editorial from the *British Medical Journal* revealed that about 160 people in England and Wales died each year from liver failure after an overdose of paracetamol. A sufficient dose seemed to reliably cause death within three to four days, and once the liver necrosis was established, it was irreversible. So here was an apparently reliable and easily available method, but how distress-ing would the death be? This was hard to gauge from the literature, but it might not be pleasant or dignified. But if the overdose of para-cetamol was followed by a large dose of sedative, the person would sleep peacefully through the liver failure. Death would take three to four days, and proper care and prevention of interference was needed during this interval.

I arranged another visit to her home, and confirmed that nothing had changed. She was still making a persistent request for assistance to end her suffering by ending her life. Her request was rational and not made under duress. I then discussed in detail the proposal for her to take an overdose of paracetamol in the evening, followed by a large dose of her sedative, and that on the following day I would admit her to hospital under my care. Her husband, acting as her medical enduring power of attorney, would refuse treatment of a presumed urinary infection and sepsis, and she would be kept comfortable until she died. I emphasised that I had no personal experience of this method, but was confident that it would cause death and if accompanied by the sedative would not cause suffering in itself. The only drawback was the time taken to die. I do not regard it as dignified for a person or their family to wait days for a certain death to be played out—the vigil can be excruciating. After prolonged discussion, she agreed to this approach and a potential date was set, to ensure that I would be available to care for her. A measure of her suffering was to be seen in her agreement to this uncertain process.

I cannot remember how I slept that night, but I waited anxiously for the phone call next morning. When it came it revealed that she had taken the paracetamol, but had been unable to take the sedative, which had been planned to follow eight hours later. However, she did not appear to be suffering unduly. I arranged her immediate admission to hospital and found her to be conscious, able to communicate that she had no pain or distress, and not obviously suffering from the lack of the sedative. Valium and morphine were ordered for palliation, and acknowledgment of her refusal of active treatment was recorded. One dose of valium was administered that evening. By the next evening, she was drowsy, had slurred speech and was difficult to understand. She had a mild fever but no evidence of jaundice, an indicator of liver failure. She became comatose overnight and died the next morning, some fifty-seven hours after ingesting the paracetamol. Despite not taking the sedative, there appeared to be no distress during this time. I had been very concerned when I learned that she had been unable to take the sedative, as I saw this as central to the relative dignity of the process. I did not simply want to enable her to die, but to ensure that she did not suffer in the process, and that her death had dignity for her and her family. I was elated when a discussion with her husband reassured me that for him that had been the case.

My elation was short-lived when I realised that I would have to complete a death certificate and a request for cremation (which required a second medical opinion). What was I going to record on this legal document—there are probably serious penalties for falsely completing such a form? I had noted during her last forty-eight hours that the movement in her right arm and hand had deteriorated markedly, and she had manifest slurred speech and drowsiness leading to coma. A stroke complicating an initial diagnosis of sepsis from a urinary tract infection was a possible explanation of her demise. Then I was shaken by an event that has never happened to me before or since—her general practitioner was providing the obligatory second signature on the cremation certificate, and he rang me to discuss the death. He must have been surprised when his patient was admitted to hospital in an emergency situation without him being contacted or consulted. I blustered through an explanation of the clinical situation, and then waited anxiously to find out whether the cremation had gone ahead. This was probably the most anxious time I have spent in the past fifteen years of helping patients to die with choice and dignity. I was very relieved when her husband rang to thank me and tell me that she had been cremated.

I had indirectly assisted Alice to hasten her death by suicide. I had given her advice and palliative support that allowed her to complete her intention to end her intolerable suffering, due to a hopeless and incurable illness. On a previous occasion, due to a lack of such advice and support, she had been thwarted and her autonomy abused. It was my intention to give her security and allow her to take control over her suffering according to her perceived best interests.

Thus ended my first deliberate assistance in dying. Perhaps I had been lucky, and to this day I have managed to avoid falsifying another death certificate. That aspect went hard with me, as I detest dishonesty, and breaking the law. How hypocritical, I hear you say, when I have presumably just broken the *Crimes Act* (which forbids assistance in suicide), to moan about falsifying a mere document. The point is that there is nothing wrong with the collection of statistical data about deaths (that does not need to be changed) but there is a great deal that is wrong with the *Crimes Act* in relation to assisting suicide.

Reading this statute, at that time, was enough to terrify me. It is not illegal for someone like Alice to end her life for rational reasons, but it is illegal to help her. This is a crude and archaic law that does not recognise the necessity for a doctor, on rare occasions, to render this assistance to a rational person for palliative reasons. It is insensitive to the needs of suffering people and forces compassionate doctors and families to break this law if they are to listen and help.

It is clear that Alice had a very different kind of illness from Betty and Len. They had terminal cancer, and pain was very prominent in their suffering, but in both cases the period of intolerable suffering was relatively short, measured in months. Sometimes it is only weeks or days. A terminal illness, such as advanced cancer, has a reasonably predictable downhill course, during which reasonable palliation of symptoms can be expected, until near the very end, when significant difficulties and a crescendo of suffering can occur.

Alice, on the other hand, had suffered progressively from MS for many years, and the end point was not even in sight. She had a hopeless illness, not a terminal illness. Most of the debate about physician–assisted dying is focused on cancer pain in terminal illness, but it is a great mistake to ignore the suffering of hopeless illness. The suffering in a hopeless illness can be far greater than in a terminal illness because of the long and uncertain time over which it will occur.

The characteristics of a hopeless illness are that:

- It is permanent with no chance of recovery, and it may have certain, remorseless progression.
- It is a severe illness causing significant unremitting symptoms.
- It has no predictable time frame.

59

- It is associated with intolerable suffering (the patient's perspective).
- There is no effective and acceptable treatment to ameliorate that suffering, or alter the course of the disease.

Thus, hopeless illness could be defined as 'an incurable illness of certain permanence or inevitable progression, whose severity causes intolerable suffering that cannot be relieved by treatment that is acceptable to the sufferer'. The fourth characteristic (intolerable suffering) is clearly subjective and dependent on the individual and his or her circumstances. What is tolerable to one person may be intolerable to another, but the person is not to be judged or condemned on those grounds. It is obviously essential that correctable factors such as treatable depression or other psychological causes or social conditions are not influencing the person's assessment of their state, but they should not be treated as someone lacking intellectual, moral or spiritual fibre simply because they find their situation intolerable. It is highly likely that the elderly and those without family and close friends may find certain conditions intolerable, but that those more supported will not. However, the interventions of well-meaning strangers may not alter such choices; rather, they should be respected.

On reflection, it was obvious that this process could have been better. The failure to ingest the sedatives might have led to problems, although I easily could have provided sedation in hospital if it had been needed (some was given). Whilst the paracetamol was successful, the time delay to death was unsatisfactory; there may have been some unrealised suffering in the process, which could be seen only as futile and essentially undignified. Moreover, the lack of a second opinion and cooperation of another doctor who knew this patient well was a problem. My ultimate feeling was that the local doctor suspected that something unusual had happened but decided to allow it to pass in the circumstances.

There had to be a better way. The Dutch had been involved with assisted dying for two decades and would surely have good information, but it was not published in the medical literature. Through a Dutch friend, I made contact with Dr Pieter Admiraal, an anaesthetist, the doyen of Dutch doctors involved with physician-assisted dying.

I now knew the optimal means, although obtaining it for patients could still be a problem. As far as finding cooperative doctors, that is still an understandable problem so long as the law remains as it is. They risk their freedom and their ability to practise their profession by becoming involved. It is surprising so many do.

Readers will observe that my actions bore little resemblance to those of Quill. No one regrets that more than I do, but our circumstances were very different. I was not Alice's treating doctor, and I felt I was running a very significant risk by getting involved at all. I did not have the ability to prescribe barbiturates for her with reasonable impunity. I did the best I could in very difficult circumstances, but recognising the inadequate outcome, I determined to do better.

7

PROLONGING LIFE

'Euthanasia is not a choice between life and death, but a choice between different ways of dying.'
Jacques Pohier (Catholic priest, excommunicated for his views on euthanasia)

On the sixth of May, 1993, I was approached by a 75-year-old woman who was severely distressed and wanted me to help her to die. She had chosen to see me because of the publicity following my inadvertent statement to the *Age* reporter in 1992.

Three months earlier, Anna Knight had appeared to be quite healthy. Since then, she had developed a bladder infection, and investigations revealed ovarian cancer that was also involving her bowel. A palliative hysterectomy (removal of womb, tubes and ovaries) was performed.

Six weeks later, having barely recovered from this procedure, she developed an acute bowel obstruction, due to the residual cancer, resulting in the removal of part of her colon. Two weeks later her bowel join leaked, resulting in a communication between the bowel and the vagina (a recto-vaginal fistula), with faeces leaking uncontrollably through the vagina. She ended up with a permanent colostomy, in lay terms, a permanent opening of the large intestine on the abdomen through which the faeces are discharged into a bag attached to the skin.

Thus, in the short space of three months, Mrs Knight had gone from an apparently normal, healthy person, through three severe abdominal operations, to someone with almost certainly incurable cancer of a most vicious kind. She had a permanent opening on her abdomen discharging faeces, which she hated and regarded as com-pletely undignified, together with a persistent discharge of pussy mucus from the rectum through the vagina, requiring the use of two pads per day. The only further treatment was the offer of chemotherapy (six courses, each lasting one month) with a possible 20 per cent chance of cure. In reality, that figure was highly optimistic, with the best chance being some palliation and a short extension of life expectancy. She was very strongly of a mind to refuse this treatment.

Not surprisingly, I found Mrs Knight to be deeply depressed, even though she was already taking antidepressants. She had been treated by a gynaecologist and a general surgeon, but she could not communi-cate with either, as one deflected her questions and anxieties while the other, although she liked him and could talk to him, simply would not acknowledge her right to self-determination. Hence, in desperation, she had found her way to me. I was confronted by a depressed, frightened woman, whose life seemed to be spiralling out of control and who, out of desperation, desired to end her life. Would I help her, she asked?

I needed to address two central questions. First, did her mental state allow her to make a rational decision and, second, was she fully informed about her medical situation? However, before embarking on a discussion of these questions, I believed it was essential to give her confidence that I would respect her opinions on end-of-life matters, and that her right to self-determination was paramount. I guaranteed my support of her right to choose. Convinced of my support, she could then discuss other issues in a calmer state of mind.

What suffering did she have that would make her want to end her life? Suffering is a personal matter, and it is not ultimately my right to judge the suffering of another, but as a doctor faced with the question of whether to assist another human being to end their life, one must make an assessment of the apparent suffering. Was it sufficient to consider giving assistance, or was there further treatment that might relieve the suffering and thus render that assistance unnecessary? Mrs Knight came to me a few days after leaving hospital following her third major abdominal operation, with a diagnosis of incurable ovarian cancer and an option to undergo chemotherapy with a highly optimistic 20 per cent chance of benefit. Moreover, she was being managed by doctors with whom she could either not communicate effectively, or who would not listen to her point of view. It was no wonder that she was severely depressed despite treatment. There is no doubt that this exogenous depression (due to external circumstances) could have a serious impact on her decisions, which could change if the depression could be relieved.

Undoubtedly, she had physical symptoms but they did not seem dominant, as she expressed them to me. She had no pain at that time, but had to deal with the irritation and discomfort of the vaginal discharge from the bowel fistula, and the care of her colostomy. The latter was more of an emotional burden than a physical one. For many people whose colostomy represents the outcome of successful treatment, its care is of little moment and it may be regarded as a boon rather than a burden. But if it is not curative, it can be seen as a bitter reminder of the disease that has brought them to this pass, and the disfigurement, odour and mess can be thoroughly hateful. This is how Mrs Knight saw her stoma and bag.

Finally, she had the knowledge that she was incurable and would decline progressively with nausea, loss of weight, pain and the ever-present possibility of another bowel obstruction to a death that she imagined would be totally undignified. For her family this would leave a memory of her that was quite unacceptable. She had existential suffering of significant proportions. Thus, to my assessment, her suffering was largely psychological, with existential and physical components.

Mrs Knight, although she had incurable cancer, was not terminally ill (that is, her time of death was not foreseeable or reasonably predictable), although she would become so. With a response from her chemotherapy, she might live for twelve to twenty-four months with a reasonable quality of life, but she did not appreciate this. I felt that if her psychological, emotional and existential suffering could be addressed, the physical components might not be sufficient to make her want to end her life. Thus the answer to my first question was that she was not in a sound state of mind to make serious decisions about her future, and with respect to the second, she was not sufficiently informed to allow appropriate decisions about treatment. The latter situation was due to difficulty in communication and the emotional turmoil associated with her illness that prevented her understanding what she needed to know. She was therefore not in a situation where any assistance to end her life could be given until these questions were addressed.

Acknowledging her right to self-determination and agreeing to help her would go a long way to relieving her anxiety and her depression. Depression is a common issue in these situations—it is vital that it be diagnosed and corrected if possible. She acknowledged that she was depressed and agreed to more aggressive antidepressant medication. There was a need to replace her negative thinking about her future with some positives, so we discussed those things that she had enjoyed doing before her operations, and I encouraged her to re-engage in these activities. I promised to talk to her treating doctors to establish a clear picture of her prognosis and likelihood of response to chemotherapy and its likely side-effects, and to inform them of her desire to be given realistic advice in the future. It is all too common that specialists treating incurable cancer paint an overly optimisticly picture regarding treatment in order to maintain 'hope', but in my experience most patients prefer realism to 'false hope'. They can ultimately accept and deal with the truth, but are bitter at being deceived. Thus I encouraged her to deal with her treating doctors in a completely open manner, and suggested that she reconsider chemotherapy, after further discussion with her oncologist on that basis. We agreed to meet again soon to continue our dialogue.

Finally, I asked her to write down her feelings about her disease, her treatment and her situation, and did so for two reasons. First, because such an exercise can be cathartic with respect to grief, guilt and anxiety, and can clear the mind of extraneous thoughts and confused thinking; and, second, because the thoughts of people in Mrs Knight's situation are not often recorded, yet they are extremely important and deserve to be part of the debate. I did not at that time appreciate how important her words were to become.

One week later, I received the first of a series of eight letters (which spanned the next sixteen months) from Mrs Knight. They formed the basis of an extensive article by journalist Nick Davies (who coined the name Anna Knight). This accompanied the statement in *The Age* by the 'Melbourne Seven' to the Premier of Victoria, admitting that they had helped patients to die.[1] The Melbourne Seven, as they became known, were a disparate and unconnected group of doctors who joined in support of a plea to change the law. None of them was charged. Some, I know, are still behaving with similar compassion.

I will let these remarkable documents speak for themselves.

13 May 1993

It was a huge relief to talk to someone who didn't reject my belief in voluntary euthanasia. It isn't just because I am in trouble that I have asked for help, it's my firm conviction that human beings have the right to say 'enough'. Eventually the law will change, but too late for many people.

Yes, I am depressed at present, and fearful, so afraid of more surgery, my abdomen was opened right down the middle three times in a little over two months, colonoscopy and gastroscopy too. I have thought of you a lot since we met, and have said a silent prayer, 'Please don't let Mr Syme be knocked down by a bus.' I would feel very much safer if you agreed to give me the information now, even if I just kept it in a safe place and didn't use it. All our lives are uncertain. My life hasn't much quality now, it's just a round of changing colostomy bags three times a day, and a repulsive job, the vaginal discharge pads need regular changing, and the fistula luckily only once a day. I don't want to eat, but push food in because I have lost 20 kilos in three months. I am almost totally deaf, 25% in one ear and none in the other, and severe tinnitus, there are these loud noises that never stop. I feel very cut off from people, no telephone, radio, group meetings, theatre, films or social occasions, and only captional TV. This all sounds very self-centred, I am telling you my story, because it explains why I feel that I have had enough of life. I am so afraid of getting into a hospital situation again where I am helpless. Once a bowel blockage started it would be too late, because nausea and vomiting are early symptoms and I couldn't keep the medication down. I am not rushing into this because I am depressed, it has been carefully thought out, if I leave it too late there could be a situation where I couldn't change my colostomy bags, and my husband couldn't do it, it's such a repulsive job that I wouldn't want him to even if he was able to. I want to avoid things like this happening; it's so easy to get into a situation where you lose control of your life. Then it's probably a long painful cancer death. I have seen this happen and it's frightening, people being kept alive to suffer, and families devastated as they watch this slow cruel death. So please let me have your information as soon as you feel able to. I won't change in my wish to control my own life, and death.

There are so many things that I want to ask you, 'How long does it take', 'Have there been failures where the person is left with mental or physical damage'—though I don't believe that you would give any information that was so risky. Last night I was kept awake for four hours with quite a bad abdominal pain, and all the time there is abdominal discomfort. Luckily all my near family agree with vol. euthanasia, my husband says that if he were in my position he would feel the same as I do, he doesn't want to watch me suffer.

So thank you again for your kindness and understanding, I will look forward to seeing you again.[2]

This letter clearly reveals the enormous relief people feel when they can communicate openly in dialogue with a doctor who respects their wishes and commits to their support. Yet there is still an anxiety about not having the medication and huge anxiety about lacking control of her life without adequate information. It also shows remarkable thought and insight into the possible outcomes, and their consequences, not only for herself but also for her family. After I phoned her daughter to deal with some of these issues, Mrs Knight sent me this letter explaining her fears.

28 July 1993

I had three operations for cancer in ten weeks, starting with a hysterectomy and large ovarian cancer, and finishing with a colostomy. The middle operation to remove more cancer was a dreadful failure because the stitches in my bowel burst. The feeling of being out of control of my body, and of my life, was distressing. A friend had recently died a long distressing cancer death; she had lived on for twelve months after the doctors had told her that there was nothing more that they could do. As I still have several pieces of inoperable cancer in my abdomen, it was easy for me to believe that this would be my fate too. Prolonged death after a lot of suffering is not unusual for cancer patients. My thoughts constantly revolved around 'How can I escape', drowning or using the car exhaust seemed to be the most available, but

I didn't have any confidence that I would be able to do either. The determination was there, but bodily weakness, not being able to involve others, or being rescued with brain damage, these thoughts were in my mind every day. One night a nurse sat with me and we talked about euthanasia, she didn't know of any nurses who were not in favour of it, and she believed that many doctors would be willing to give their patients this release from hopeless suffering. I left the hospital deeply depressed and with my mind full of fear, three months later the depression has lifted but the anxiety and fear are still there. I told one doctor that the law re euthanasia was not civilized, and his reply was that euthanasia and civilization did not go hand in hand. He said that the doctors now give their patients a good quality of life, and at the end a peaceful and dignified death. I wasn't rude enough to say, 'Don't talk such rot', but that is what I was thinking. If I had not felt so weak and helpless perhaps I would have had the spirit to argue. In some cases doctors may give their patients release at the end, but only after a lot of physical and mental distress, and not in the majority of cases. What the doctor sees as a good quality of life can be quite different from how the patient feels, doctors don't see the daily miseries, and the struggle with weakness that many people face every day. Our bodies belong to us, and the law should not deprive us of the assistance of our doctors if living becomes intolerable; we have needed their help to live, and now we need their help to die.

These letters convinced me that she badly needed the information and the drugs to give her control over her future life, and to eliminate the fear and toxic anxiety verging on terror that were obviously dominating her waking moments. So when I saw her next, I discussed the medication that she would need to end her life, namely a lethal quantity of barbiturates. Since the publicity of 1992, I was very concerned about writing a prescription for barbiturates myself, so I suggested she seek them from her general practitioner, with whom she had had a long and friendly relationship.

There is very good evidence that terminally ill people who acquire the medication that would allow them to end their lives, should they wish, actually live longer and better as a result, whether or not they need to take the medication. We also discussed the value of chemotherapy, and I emphasised that she could try it and cease it at any time if she felt the side effects were too distressing. I did not discuss the technicalities of using barbiturates at this stage, as I wanted to be sure she would consult with me again before considering their use.

I don't expect you to answer this, but I find it easier to tell you how I am thinking this way as I can't use the phone. My doctor who has known me for over twenty years has given me a prescription for 100 Soneryl 100 mg with one repeat. Then because she thought that Soneryl may have been taken off the market she also gave me a NeurAmyl (100) 50 mg script with one repeat. She has always known me to be a rational person, and I feel bad about deceiving her by asking for them as sleeping tablets, but my husband and daughter both assure me that she would not have been deceived for one minute; she knew exactly what she was doing. I have been doing a great deal of thinking, and I know that you are right when you say that timing is important and that I am not ready yet. Your advice has helped me greatly, and I want to talk with you again because you will help me to get some of the things that are worrying me into the right perspective. One problem is that if I wait for long I may become ill and unable to do it alone, or a bowel blockage may stop the medication from getting into my intestines. The thought of dying with no one beside me, or even knowing, really makes me afraid. My husband completely agrees with me about taking this way of avoiding what could be a long drawn out, a painful cancer death, but he doesn't want to know just when, so he can't help me. Our daughter is willing, but I want to protect her from such a traumatic experience. So I must do it while I am well enough to cope, and be careful of all the important details. Will I have enough, now I am scared by the thought. Another reason for me to fear becoming ill is that there isn't anyone to change my colostomy bag, my husband couldn't do it, and as it fills up at different times each day, the district nurse isn't the answer; I still hate that colostomy. All the people that I have read about who die from overdoses seem to near the end anyhow, and they have suffered a great deal of pain and had chemotherapy, and had help. Is it wrong of me to wish to avoid going through all that mental distress and pain by doing it before I reach that stage? Writing all this and knowing that you will read it with kindness and understanding has eased my mind. It will be a very difficult thing to do. Am I brave enough?

How pleased I was that she had obtained the necessary dose of barbiturates, yet she still had desperate anxieties about the technical details. It was clearly time for the dialogue to continue, but this letter demonstrates perfectly how the clandestine nature of this sort of illegal help does not totally allay the fears and anxieties of patients. She was fearful of involving her family, fearful of dying alone, fearful of missing her opportunity and fearful of making a mess of it. Yet some say that suicide is the coward's way—I don't believe it. It takes real courage to confront your illness and destiny and take control of both. Perhaps that is why many patients want the doctor to deliver the fatal dose. Yet the responsibility for such an important decision lies rightly with the suffering person, and there is no more powerful demonstration of their need and intent than their own action.

28 July 1993

This is to let you know that I have started chemotherapy, the reason for my change of mind was the wish to care for my husband for as long as possible, it seemed selfish to refuse anything that may keep me living for a bit longer. I think of you very often, and always with warmth and gratitude. When I left the hospital I felt so afraid and desperate, it was an enormous relief for me to talk freely to you about my beliefs and fears. I left you feeling 'safer', your wise counselling reassured me that it wasn't unreasonable to think about self-deliverance, but that it must never be a premature act, it must be a rational decision, made when my condition became intolerable and I no longer had the will to live. When I think of my lonely room and my little bottle of barbiturates, I feel fear to die alone with no one to hold my hand and give me courage; that is a very frightening thought. The alternative of living on through months or perhaps years of physical and mental deterioration, with my much loved family helplessly watching as I slowly die; that is a dreadful thought too. The present laws relating to euthanasia are not humane, they must be changed. We need some brave and compassionate politicians who will admit this, and actively work towards getting the changes made. As the law stands thousands of people are condemned to prolonged and hopeless suffering. Politicians have bodies too, and the day may come when they are caught in this inhumane dying trap, then they may well think 'Why didn't I act while I had some influence?' Doctors don't usually want to talk about any form of euthanasia; they can't legally help, not even in a stand-by capacity. Many would be willing and caring enough to assist with their patients' dying, just as they have given their professional help during their living years. It's when people are facing death that they most need doctor's support and guidance. To try, and fail, that is a fear that people feel. In some cases after the patient has been through a lot of hopeless suffering they are allowed to die, but that's not good enough. The desperation and the longing for a peaceful death that many people are forced to go through isn't humane, it's cruelty.

Fear, weakness and pain can rob even a brave person of their courage and dignity, and knowing that their families last memory of them will be of a slowly disintegrating, dependent and probably frightened object in a bed must often cause acute distress. Good memories can be cancelled out by a prolonged and dreadful death.

What an advocate! If only the voices of those with intolerable suffering could be heard more frequently in this debate. What I did note in this letter was a more positive attitude and an alleviation of her depression. This was evident in her decision to proceed with chemotherapy, and in finding a purpose in her life; that is, in continuing to look after her husband. These benefits are gained by being able to communicate openly and in obtaining medication that places the sufferer in control.

23 October 1993

This is to let you know what has been happening to me. You gave me help when I needed it badly, and I want to keep in contact. The fourth chemo treatment is over, and the only really bad effect is that it has caused a further hearing loss. There is tiredness, poor appetite, and a few other things, but I had to have chemo because to go down without even trying to extend my life would have been selfish; my husband needs me. I still want it to be over because of the possibility of a long downhill slide, with weakness and dependence on others really scares me. Loss of dignity is worse than pain, and colostomies are undignified. Using my medication and releasing myself from life would avoid a long drawn out death, but I must be sure that doing this won't hurt my family. They could accept it more easily if I am in obvious pain and distress, but if I waited until then I may not manage it successfully, taking pain-killers may interfere with the action of the medication, or I may be confused and mess it up. Will just have to wait and let events unfold. Yesterday my husband and I visited a funeral director and made advance arrangements; it didn't seem a morbid thing to do. We went to the Cemetery too, and there is a place under a beautiful old gum tree where ashes can be put directly into the ground amongst the roots, they place a small boulder over the ashes. The tree has a silver grey trunk and large spreading arms. A feeling of peace came to me beneath that tree, I felt ready to let go and become part of the earth, but with a healthy husband standing beside me there was also a reason to keep on living.

Since I had not seen Mrs Knight for some months, I wrote to her as follows:

Dear Mrs Knight,

Thank you for your note. I am pleased that you have had the chemotherapy without any very significant problems. I can sense some anxieties coming through in your letter, and can only say that if at any time you want to come and see me and talk about these, and gain some further insight into your problem, I would be only too happy to see you.

5 December 1993

Thank you for your letter; you were right when you sensed that I still feel some anxiety, but I am coping with this reasonably well. Self-doubt is the main cause, I want to go through this cancer experience, and eventually death, with courage, and want to protect my family as much as possible … It was like being on a conveyor belt, the loss of dignity was worse than the pain. I felt helpless. Now I try not to look into the future, but some fear and anxiety are always there. I will never use my barbiturates while my husband is alive, unless my situation is really bad, and will come to you first for your counselling. Just knowing that you are there is a comfort.

We did meet again and discussed her future in further detail. She clearly had ongoing anxieties but, with support, felt able to carry on. Her initial depression had gone, to be replaced by anxiety, which I did my best to minimise by continued encouragement and support.

26 August 1994

If I could come and talk with you sometime I will be relieved and grateful. I have kept on struggling to regain some health, but each operation has left me weaker and with less joy in living. Six weeks ago, my surgeon shifted my stoma from the right to the left side. This operation was supposed to make me more comfortable, but it has not been a success. My colon had become stuck together and the surgeon only had a small free piece, which had to be stretched across my abdomen, so a good stoma could not be formed. Now the stitched part has been pulled back inside me by the tight colon, this causes me pain every day, and I can't take a large enough dose of MS Contin [morphine] to relieve this because Contin makes my faeces too firm, and this pushes the wafer away from my abdomen and faeces spread everywhere. We are trying to get a balance between the Contin and a faecal softener. Another distressing thing is a mucous discharge from my rectum that I can't control; even a little causes a painful bearing down feeling. I am trying to control this with suppositories. Enemas are no help because my weak rectal muscles won't let the enema fluid stay in. I feel weak; it's not easy to eat, and I am tired of this roller coaster of pain, surgery, and fear of what will go wrong next. I am telling you all this so that you won't think that I am a wimp who has given in easily, now I feel it's getting close to the time when I will decide to take my barbiturates, and I want to do this while I am still strong enough to do it all myself. All the adult members of my family agree with and support voluntary euthanasia. I may have to use a plastic bag to be sure of a quick death, but I would like to avoid this as it may be more upsetting for my family. Still better that than try and fail; that is my big fear.

This letter made it clear to me that she was finding it difficult to continue because of severe anxiety about how to use her medication, and fear of failure. Such anxiety can utterly erode any remaining quality of life and, in certain circumstances, lead to premature and irrational suicide. She now needed clear advice on the use of her medication and reassurance as to its efficacy.

9 September 1994

I feel very weak and shaky today, and feel that I must act soon or a nursing home will get me. These are a few questions I hope that you will answer.

I haven't any Zofran tabs (anti-emetic); I have Maxolon and Zadine. My surgeon said that Zofran can only be prescribed with chemotherapy. So is there another anti-emetic that a doctor will prescribe that will do?

My weight is now only 53 kg, and I am losing each week so is it still all right to take 10 mg of Soneryl (100 tabs); no doubt I will lose some more in the next few weeks.

Do many people take enough medication and fail to die, this worries me?

I sometimes feel that I am imposing on you in my need for support and advice. I am always grateful, and hope that you will reply quickly because I can feel my strength going and it does take strength to get all the arrangements made properly.

We met after this letter and I dispelled any suggestion that she would need to use a bag over her head. Whilst a bag over the head to exclude oxygen, causing death by hypoxia, is effective, it is not tolerable without a large dose of sedatives to cause deep sleep and prevent the unpleasant symptoms of excess carbon dioxide. More importantly, although it is efficient, the vast majority of people find this concept quite undignified, and they do not want to leave such a lasting memory. I reassured her that her dose of barbiturates was quite sufficient and reliable on its own—there is no doubt that the spectre of taking medication and not being successful causes severe anxiety to many hopelessly ill people. They need certainty that the action that they are taking will be secure and that they will die with dignity. The use of an appropriate dose of barbiturates provides this, allowing the person to say goodbye to their family and friends, and then go quietly to sleep in five to thirty minutes, and die in one half to two hours and often less, but with occasional exceptions where death takes longer.

14 October 1994

This is the letter that I gave to my doctor and she was very firm that 'yes', she would honour it, and talk to her colleagues too. Wish that I could write more, and express myself better. I am feeling fear, not of death, but of failing to die. It would be wonderful to have a doctor standing by.

Each day is full of weakness and nausea, every mouthful has to be pushed in, this isn't living, it's slow dying. I am still afraid, I don't want to do this to myself, but how I long to die—quickly.

To any doctor who is attending me,

If I have any bodily or mental ailment, or I am found in any life threatening condition, then I am asking the attending doctor not to try resuscitation or send me to hospital. Please let me die in our own home, peacefully and without pain. I have terminal cancer, ovarian Stage 3; this may have spread further now as I feel weak and ill. I also have a colostomy which has not been a success, this causes distress and pain every day. I have had four operations in eighteen months, it's been downhill all the way and I can only expect this to continue that way. I am old and *ready to die*. This is a rational decision made after a lot of thought. Also I am almost totally deaf with loud continuous tinnitus, there isn't any peace. If I do linger on, please ask a nurse to come in, the colostomy will need attention. Bethlehem have kept in touch (palliative care) for eighteen months. *Please* don't take away my chance to die peacefully. I may need pain relief, but I don't want anything that will save my life. *I want to die.*

15 October 1994

I feel dreadful today, eating is punishment. You have been so kind and patient. I don't know today whether I will take my medication on Sunday night, but how I want to. My only fear is of failure, not of dying. Regrets of course; I think of that last look at my family's faces; it's hard to do that.

Her daughter rang me shortly after this to say she had died peacefully. She did not die alone. She had been able to say goodbye to her loved ones, an enormously important issue. She could achieve this because she had gained control over the timing of her death.

Because she knew when she would die, she was able to say goodbye, to find closure to her life, to ensure that all those things that needed to be said to her significant friends and family were addressed. A sudden death is sometimes considered to be a good death, no lingering or prolonged suffering, but for those left behind, there is an exaggerated sense of loss in a sudden, unexpected departure. Yet, today, many people take their lives alone for fear that the presence of their family will put them in danger of prosecution for assisting in their suicide. And by failing to address the issue of rational suicide, our parliamentarians condemn many terminal and/or hopelessly ill people like Diane and Mrs Knight to die alone. Our parliamentarians are so afraid to address physician-assisted dying that they cannot even reassure people that they will not be in breach of the law if they are merely present for support and to say good-bye to a loved one who is taking her life to end suffering! The lack of this security led Dr Philip Nitschke to organise twenty-one brave people to be with Nancy Crick when she took her life on the Gold Coast in May 2001 in order to test the law. Two years after Crick's suicide, the Queensland Police Commissioner finally announced that none of the twenty-one was to be prosecuted because of a lack of evidence. He did, however, have the consideration to declare: 'Being present when someone takes their own life does not in itself constitute an offence'.

Was Mrs Knight unusual in choosing to end her life in order to end her suffering? Not at all. Palliative care experts acknowledge that 'Suicide was openly discussed as an option by over a quarter of these patients (with severe symptoms) … only a particularly severe degree of overall fatigue appeared to distinguish those patients who endorsed suicide as an option.'[3] Roger Hunt's palliative care group in Adelaide found that of 331 patients who died in their hospice, 11 per cent expressed the view 'I wish it would hurry up'; 6 per cent said, 'could you hurry it up'; and 6 per cent said, 'please do something now'.[4] British researchers Seale and Addington-Hall found in a large survey of 3696 people who were dying or had died that 28 per cent of those in hospice (palliative care) reported that earlier death would have been better. Twenty-six per cent of those who died had stated they wanted an earlier death, and 7.9 per cent of the deceased had wanted euthanasia.[5]

As I write this some thirteen years later, I am struck by the continuing level of anxiety described by Mrs Knight in her letters. Although I gave her my strong reassurance that I would support her, and subsequently gave her information as to what drugs she needed, she remained with unrelieved anxiety. Even obtaining the drugs from her general practitioner did not fully alleviate her psychological distress. It was not enough control to allow peace of mind and to allow her to obtain the

best possible palliation. It was not until she had the complete information as to how to use the drugs in detail that she was more reassured
and relaxed. I did not sufficiently appreciate this at the time, as I
was concerned that she might have taken a pre-emptive action and was
quite worried about the legality of my actions and the consequences
that might follow.

I had provided Mrs Knight with support and advice (not medication) that assisted her to end her life. She did this after a prolonged
struggle with pain, indignity, fear and anxiety. My intention was to give
her control over her circumstances, to help her to go as far as she could
on life's journey, but ultimately allow her to express her intention to
end her suffering. Did I provide Mrs Knight with illegal assistance in
suicide by this dialogue and advice? This question occupied my mind
more strongly after my next end-of-life encounter.

8

THE NATURE OF SUFFERING

'I would like death to come to me while I am planting cabbages, caring little for death and even less for the imperfections of my garden.'
Michel de Montaigne (1533–1592), French essayist and philosopher

Most people, in this covert era, are diffident or embarrassed about approaching their medical practitioner for medical advice and assistance in ending their own life. They usually make a tentative initial contact by telephone and less often by letter, but some actually make an appointment with a doctor to discuss the matter. The initial telephone call provides a limited opportunity to assess the detail and context of the request and allows some space to think about the issues and the appropriate response before meeting such a person across the consulting desk. A letter also creates this space, in fact more space, but provides somewhat less basis for decision-making because it is not interactive and only a limited amount of information may be available. Nevertheless, both these approaches give the doctor time to decide whether it is appropriate to become involved and in what way, whereas the direct consultation is a good deal more challenging.

Margaret adopted the consultation approach. I did not recognise her name on my appointment list, nor did I know her referring doctor. This always suggests the potential for an interesting or unusual problem. Obviously a new patient with a new problem, but could it be for a second opinion, or about an unmentionable problem? In fact there was no referral letter from her doctor. When I met Margaret in the waiting room I found a frail, elderly woman sitting in a wheelchair. She was obviously unable to move the wheelchair herself, indicating that her upper arms were weak. I greeted her and pushed her chair into the consulting room, already sensing that a request for assistance to die was in the offing. My response to such a situation is always ambivalent. On the one hand it may provide an opportunity for really valuable and rewarding service. At the same time there is an element of risk and difficulty about these matters that means that a very demanding process is about to begin, which will require the very best medical care that I can summon.

Margaret had probably suffered from motor neurone disease (MND) since 1990, but the diagnosis had not been made until 1992. There initially had been some weakness in her right leg, which caused her to fall and break her right ankle. In 1992 she had spinal surgery for this weakness with negligible improvement but she was left with back pain. Following this, the diagnosis of MND became clear, with all the serious implications this has for any individual. MND is a disease of the nervous system of unknown cause that tends to affect people in middle and older age. It is a condition of relentless and relatively rapid progression, such that the time from onset to death is rarely more than five years and often a good deal less. It causes progressive paralysis of the limbs and, usually in the later stages, of the muscles involved in swallowing, speaking and breathing. Variants can occur, when the initial onset can affect the muscles of breathing, or of swallowing and talking. There is absolutely no treatment available and the disease progresses inevitably to total paralysis and dependence. The increasing difficulty in swallowing can lead to inhalation of food and saliva, fits of coughing and potential airway obstruction; at the same time, progressive difficulty in breathing leads to either death by lack of oxygen or the need for artificial respiration. The inability to swallow will also lead, if it is accepted, to the placement of a feeding tube through the abdominal wall into the stomach (PEG) to prevent death by dehydration and starvation, as eating becomes not only impossible but also dangerous. A further difficulty is weakening of the voice and trouble with communication. Tragically, it leaves the intellect untouched while destroying the body. For someone who lives almost entirely through the mind, like the great physicist Stephen Hawking, this disease may be endured with artificial support of both breathing and nutrition, but for most people it creates an intolerable situation.

My first task was to establish the status of Margaret's illness. She told me that she was now barely able to walk and used a wheelchair for any significant movement but she could not propel herself. Thus she had lost the effective use of her legs and had almost lost the function in her right arm and hand, although she was still just able to sign her own name. The function in her left arm and hand was quite good. She was able to live in her own home with help, and she had been pleased that her grand-daughter had been able to come to live with her. Her bladder function was good apart from some slight urgency, but this did create a problem since her ability to get quickly to the toilet was limited. This posed a significant potential threat, because urinary incontinence is one of the most feared challenges to human dignity. Any urologist can confirm a woman's dread of loss of urinary control. She was obviously extremely emotionally labile during the course of this dialogue, and broke into tears on a number of occasions as she related her story. What made matters even worse for her was the recent loss of her husband. He had had a stroke in 1991, which had left him with partial paralysis but, more importantly, complete loss of memory. Despite her own impairment, Margaret had looked after her husband in this condition for some three and a half years, but in January of 1995 he had died. In one sense this was a relief because she was finding it increasingly difficult to help him, but it also represented a loss of her beloved partner of fifty-four years and robbed her of one of the foundations of her reason for living.

Margaret had come to ask me for assistance to help her to die, but not yet. I had complete empathy with this request and told her so. I indicated that I would give her my support to that end. There are some circumstances and conditions under which it is not easy to reach a decision to help people in this way, but I have no difficulty in coming to this conclusion with sufferers of MND. It is arguably the worst physical condition that anybody can be afflicted with. Not only is the disease incredibly disabling physically but the psychological and existential distress is also enormous. The progressive loss of motor function means that persons who might wish to take their own life may eventually, through paralysis, be rendered completely unable to do so and become dependent on others for this help. If they are to act to help themselves then they must act before they lose hand function and may face having to end their life before they would otherwise wish to do so. The loss of hand function and the ability to swallow may force the sufferer into a pre-emptive action, unless they are to rely on the assistance of another. There was absolutely no doubt that Margaret, having reached a fairly advanced stage of this disease and having lost her husband, was firmly committed to ending her life before it went to its natural conclusion, when she would be faced with a state of total dependence and reliance on tube feeding and respiratory support by a machine. In that event she would need someone to wipe her bottom and would not even have the small consolation of tasting her own food.

Having established the nature of her disease and her clear and precise wish not to allow the disease to take its natural course, and having provided a declaration of respect for her choice and my practical support, I next had to consider just how I would be able to assist her.

Assistance in this regard, in my mind, involves two things. First, it involves doing everything possible to ensure that the suffering each person has is minimised, and providing support to make the person's remaining life as rewarding as possible. Second, it involves devising a suitable means by which such patients can end their life at the right time—the time when they deem it appropriate. There is no doubt that many people who are given a diagnosis of terminal illness and who have suffering that is relentless, severe and untreatable will get depressed. It may be the case, however, that unless the physical and psychological circumstances can be changed that the treatment of depression will fail. It is imperative to do the utmost to relieve any physical symptoms that may be present, but just as important to try to find some activities that the person is still capable of doing that can provide some sense of achievement and purpose. A life without purpose is depressing.

Margaret was not suffering any significant pain at this point in her illness but was certainly emotionally labile and possibly suffering from a depressed mood. The question of depression is a relative one; a balance between the change in emotional state and the degree of suffering (actual and potential) caused by the disease. A depressed mood for somebody in her circumstances would not be at all surprising and is not necessarily or easily affected by antidepressant medication. In my view, her mood was not out of balance with her disease state and would be very likely to be improved by my reassurance and support rather than by antidepressant drugs. It was impossible to do anything about her paralysis, but I did attempt to find out what things she could do and what would provide her with some satisfaction. She had always been a keen reader and writer. She was still able to use a keyboard, so I encouraged her to set down her thoughts about her illness, to describe her feelings, and in fact to create a progressive diary as things evolved.

Margaret was taking no medications and would therefore need to obtain some drugs if she was to be able to take her own life. She had a copy of 'Departing Drugs', a Canadian manual giving information about medications that might be useful and advice as to how to take them, including a description of the use of a bag to create hypoxia (lack of oxygen) after taking a sedative. Although I was not impressed with the dignity of this method, she was quite comfortable with using it.

I was relieved not to have to prescribe any medication personally, but assured her that, if properly employed, the plastic bag method was highly reliable. We discussed this concept in detail, and I indicated to her which simple sedatives would be best to obtain from her general practitioner. I once again gave her my commitment to assist and support her and arranged to see her again in a few weeks.

Within a few days I received from Margaret copies of three notes that she had written at an earlier time. On 13 March 1992, shortly after she had been given the diagnosis of MND, she wrote as follows:

> There is in this place a woman sentenced to death. Here she sits, head in hand, pondering. Soft chirruping of night insects, low noise of distant traffic, murmur of sea and dark silhouette of nearby trees, palpable living entities encompass her. After her ceasing these will go on. How much longer will fingers be able to grasp biro to communicate thoughts? How much longer will the body support the functioning mind?

The second note was dated 7 January 1995:

> So nearly three years has gone by since the woman last decided to commit her thoughts to paper. Then she was in Manly and had only known of her fatal disease for a few months. Incredulity had given way to the reality of the slow inevitable disintegration of her body that she was destined to witness whilst she remained in full possession of her faculties. Rage and devastating tears were still with her, less frequently now. Somehow she was summoning some inner strength and was coping with a legally blind husband, who since his stroke three and half years ago now walked with a stick and suffered a total memory loss of all events since his childhood. How was she to cope with this further burden of her gradually increasing debility? She was her husband's carer, who was to be hers?

Reflecting on this note, she wrote on 30 April 1995:

What a great change has taken place over my life since I wrote those words! Bill died on the twentieth of January—just one month after his 87th birthday. Previous to his stroke we had an agreement that if either of us were either mentally or physically disabled the other would take the necessary steps to ensure that the other's life would not be unduly prolonged; but his stroke had resulted in a personality change for Bill—he became euphoric. I could not talk to him seriously about my diagnosis. He could not understand its implications for us both and if I did get through to him he could not discuss any possible solutions. If I did manage to communicate with him it would all vanish after his next sleep. As he drifted more and more into his limited world with only brief flashes of the old Bill, his general health also deteriorated until he was sleeping most of the time. I cherish the times we sat together, me in my wheelchair pulled up to the arm of his easy chair so that we could hold hands and thus silently experience that affinity we had that needed no vocal expression.

So my partner of nearly fifty-four years is dead and I am left to cope with a desolate future. None of them [her family] in a position to offer permanent care; in any case I would not wish any of them to be burdened with that responsibility. How can I occupy myself? One hand the right almost useless and the left arm and hand slowly going the same way. Unable to stand unaided, barely able to toilet myself or get into or out of bed, unable to move freely in the bed, difficulty in using cutlery and this is only the beginning. How much longer must I travel this demoralising path?

A further note, written almost two weeks before she first saw me, was dated 7 March 1995:

I didn't ask to be created and I certainly had no hand in giving my body Motor Neurone Disease surely as an individual I should at least be able to say when I have had enough of this life. To watch one's abilities grow weaker each day knowing there is no cure and no way to reverse the process until you become a helpless heap of flesh unable to move, unable to speak, unable to swallow, yet still in possession of all your mental faculties is surely a condition of supreme human misery. A person who helps a victim of this disease to die while they still have some semblance of human dignity can only be seen as someone having great human compassion.

One week after she first saw me, she wrote:

I have felt much better able to face the days ahead since talking with you. The ever present fear of being looked after in some establishment not of my choosing had been driving me into an uncontrollable depression stripping me of any motive to get on with some kind of meaningful action. At least I am now using this difficult machine which has a mind of its own especially designed to exasperate anyone over the age of ten.

When I saw Margaret again on 26 April, the most obvious change was in her demeanour. Whereas she had previously been tearful and afraid, now she was more confident and relaxed. Her state of weakness had altered only slightly. I again discussed her views regarding the future and she was adamant that she did not want to go into nursing home care; when she could no longer manage in her own home, she clearly wished to end her own life. Nor would she accept the insertion of an artificial feeding tube or the use of artificial respiration. She had obtained a quantity of sedatives, and would be able to obtain more, but these would not in themselves be fatal. She would clearly need, because of her paralysis, help to pulverise the tablets and mix the powder with a sweet substance so that she could ingest the dose quickly. Once she was asleep, she would need assistance to place a plastic bag over her head to create fatal hypoxia. The sleeping dose would be effective only in making her unaware of any unpleasant sensations while she died of lack of oxygen. So her next need was for clear and open communication with members of her family, or others whom she could trust, to ensure that they fully understood her present suffering and how it would progress, and exactly what she wanted to do about it. She already had a sound understanding of her disease and how it would progress, and she had established communication with her medical practitioner. Now she had to continue that communication within her family.

Margaret wrote to me again on 26 May:

Thank you very much for seeing me again and discussing my problems with me. It is a great comfort to talk to someone who is sympathetic to your point of view and suggests a constructive course of action … I have been prescribed Mogadon for my sleeplessness … I have also contacted the Buddhist institute and hope to start meditation again and I had a holiday in the country with a friend … I am striving to make my life worthwhile but each week sees me gradually deteriorating; my right arm hardly functions, my right hand barely writes a signature, my left leg has to be lifted around and my carer can just transfer me to the car and the shower. This is all accompanied by stiffness, soreness in joints, ringing in ears, inability to sit up properly and lack of sleep while I contemplate the lingering horrors to come.

It was not easy for Margaret to get out and about, so I left any further visit to her discretion while asking her to come and see me or contact me at any time that she felt it would help her. She arranged to see me again on 12 July. By this time there had been further deterioration, particularly in her left arm. She had now arranged for 24-hour care in her apartment and was very content with that arrangement—'they are supportive interesting women who are willing to share their lives and thoughts with me and we have developed a happy rapport'. We again discussed her attitude, which had not changed. I made sure that she was completely conversant with what she needed to do in order to take control of her life and death.

Margaret's final letter to me was dated 10 October 1995:

Thank you for your letter sent some weeks ago. I have not replied earlier because I have not had a computer. My left hand, although worse is still able to manage the keys. My right hand is pretty well useless. I can no longer stand unaided nor can I sit up unaided. I can still feed myself although swallowing is occasionally a problem. My breathing is shallow and speaking is tiring and sometimes indistinct and hard to hear. As we both knew life is becoming increasingly difficult and hopeless.

I spent four days in palliative care at the request of my neurologist in order to look into my depression and establish a regime of appropriate medication. It was an experience never to be repeated. I am not taking the antidepressant prescribed, because I do not feel any need to.

Thank you once again for your willingness to give me support when I need it most.

Margaret's comments on palliative care are interesting. While palliative care conveys many benefits to many people, it is not the answer for everyone. It stresses its intention to respect the decisions of those for whom it cares, but it does have a philosophy that challenges people who express a wish to end their life by active means. It assumes that such people have either unrelieved suffering and unrecognised depression, or social or spiritual problems that are unresolved. They may feel they are being treated as an intellectual or moral pygmy as the multi-disciplinary team descends upon them to resolve these presumed problems. The invasive nature of palliative care is not intended but is difficult to avoid in any highly organised system of care. It does not appeal to those who prefer to control their own medical care, preferably on a one-to-one basis. Margaret's comments on her depression and antidepressant medication were penetrating. I think she was affirming that, for her, the reassurance she had received from me and the sense of control she had achieved were infinitely more valuable than antidepressant medication and cloying institutional palliative care.

I made a comment earlier on the significance of incontinence, particularly for women. Here is one intolerable symptom for which there are a variety of methods of potential solution. No one method is necessarily superior to another. The intention of all those methods is relief from that intolerable symptom. One common outcome may be reached in a variety of ways. This is not uncommon in medicine. Should the relief of terminal or hopeless suffering be any different? Palliative care alone cannot be the solution for everyone.

Enclosed with the letter Margaret referred to was a small quantity of anti-emetic tablets to prevent the possibility of vomiting when she took her sedative dose. Sensing that she would not be able to cope much longer, I rang her for a final chat. She was calm and she was ready. She was grateful for the support, and the advice she had obtained had relieved her numbing anxiety and allowed her to live longer and to live better as a result.

I received a phone call in my rooms on the morning of 14 November from a woman who identified herself as one of Margaret's carers to tell me that she had died the previous night and that the tablets had worked perfectly. I was pleased to know Margaret had found a peaceful death, but somewhat alarmed that someone I did not know apparently had significant knowledge of what had taken place. I was sure Margaret knew the gravity of the charge of assisting in suicide, but did the carer? I could but await the outcome.

It was obvious the cat was out of the bag when I received a request from the Homicide Squad on 14 March 1996 for a statement about my relationship with Margaret, in order to assist the coroner, who eventually held an inquest more than a year later. Apparently Margaret had made no secret of the fact she had intended to take her own life, and left an audiotape exonerating anyone else from involvement in her death. Her doctor certified her death as due to MND and she was cremated, but her carer, a few days later, recounted the story to two friends, one of whom reported it to the police. The coroner found Margaret had made a rational decision to end her life using information from the booklet 'Departing Drugs', but believed that because of her paralysed state she would not have been able to achieve this alone. The coroner found her carer had contributed to her death by purchasing apple puree (to mix with the powdered sedative) and her daughter had contributed to her death by placing a plastic bag over her head. Despite these clear findings, the Director of Public Prosecutions took no further action.

As with Mrs Knight, I had provided Margaret with advice and support, and also assistance with non-lethal medication (an anti-emetic). Margaret chose her own method of self-deliverance and I am sure she would have done so even without my help, probably much sooner and with considerably more distress. I am convinced my assistance allowed her to live longer and to live better.

Dr Walter Kade, an Oregon general practitioner, had been opposed to the Oregon legislation of 1997 that allowed a doctor to prescribe lethal medication for self-administration to terminally ill patients. He wrote about his first experience of such a request by one of his patients, whom he knew very well. She was a young woman dying, after ten years of treatment, from a blood cancer (lymphoma). Although initially resistant, he did, after an intense dialogue, help her. His comments on this experience are very pertinent:

> I have also redefined intolerable suffering. I now believe that it may occur in ways quite different from those we as physicians normally consider and that intolerable suffering is best defined by the patient. My patient was suffering at the core of her being without agonising pain, anorexia or night sweats. She had become

increasingly dependent on others for virtually all activities. Her dignity, her self-esteem had been stripped away. The vitality of her being had passed. Yes, her life, as she defined it, had become futile. Finally, I have also accepted that my emotional turmoil in great part reflected my entrance into uncharted territory for physicians. Although we have accepted our roles as comforters in end-of-life care, we have not struggled with or found solutions to active roles in aiding patients in accomplishing their deaths. I am grateful for the great disruption in my emotional stability that this experience precipitated. This act should never be easy, never routine. It should be among the most difficult and disquieting acts we embark upon.[1]

Most doctors are able to relate to extreme physical suffering but may not, without open dialogue, be aware of the subtler forms of suffering, or may think that they are not of medical consequence. My dialogues with Alice, Mrs Knight and Margaret had led me to a deeper understanding of suffering. Whilst they all had physical problems—pain and paralysis—it was very clear that a major part of their suffering was psychological and existential. The extreme anxiety of having no control was palpable in each of their letters, and the profound effect of burden, dependence and loss of meaning and purpose was very clear.

9

TERMINAL SEDATION

'The easing of death, as an intentional double effect, is common place
in palliative care and general practice.'[1]
Jessica Corner, Director and Deputy Dean (Nursing), Centre for
Cancer and Palliative Care Studies, Royal Marsden Hospital

In early 1995, I was carrying out some research into the varying rates of progression of prostate cancer, with or without different forms of hormonal treatment. This involved studying the file of every patient whom I had treated for prostate cancer over the previous seven years. In June 1989, I had seen a 56-year-old man who was describing some moderate difficulty in urinating, together with pain in the right lower ribs. My examination revealed some suspiciously enlarged lymph glands in the left side of his neck and a tender rib. His prostate gland was enlarged though not obviously cancerous, but his PSA test, a blood test to detect the possibility of prostate cancer, was elevated to an extent that made a diagnosis of disseminated prostate cancer certain. He had incurable prostate cancer with extensive spread. Hormonal treatment was commenced (non-curative, but designed to slow the progress of his cancer and hopefully provide palliation of his symptoms), which was remarkably successful with his symptoms abating and his PSA test falling to normal over the next six months.

This spectacular remission continued for three years until my patient began to develop pain in various parts of his skeleton, and a bone scan confirmed widespread dissemination of cancer. Pain was felt particularly in both thighs, right groin and lumbar spine. By February 1994 his symptoms were accelerating and he was admitted to a teaching hospital with incipient paraplegia (paralysis and loss of feeling in the lower limbs) due to cancer in his spine. This catastrophe was averted by a spinal operation, but within three months he was readmitted when his right thigh bone fractured (due to the cancer), and a further palliative operation was performed. When I last saw him in April 1994, he was slowly deteriorating with weight loss, poor appetite and loss of energy, the typical manner of decline for prostate cancer. Further radiotherapy had had little effect on groin and back pain; he was taking oral morphine and had started in palliative care. At this point I lost track of his progress. I did receive a summary of his last admission to hospital where he had died with what was described as 'good symptom control'.

To complete my research information on him, I obtained the man's file (in 1997) from the teaching hospital where he had been admitted for his terminal medical care on 5 July 1994. His death summary at the front of his medical record described how his disease had progressed, how he had been confined to a wheelchair by the onset of complete paraplegia and had developed escalating back pain that was not being controlled by oral morphine. The death summary recorded that he 'was admitted and commenced on a subcutaneous morphine and maxolon [an anti-emetic] infusion to control his pain. He continued to be agitated and distressed, however good symptom control was achieved by increasing his morphine and adding some midazolam [a sedative] to his infusion'.

He died on 15 July, ten days after admission.

This death summary suggested a relatively benign and well controlled management of this patient's terminal illness, but when I looked
into the detailed record, particularly to the nursing notes, an entirely
different picture emerged. The examining doctor found that he had no
sensation or movement in his legs and had a distended bladder due to
paralysis of his bladder muscle, all due to the sudden interference of
nerve supply by the spinal cancer. He was pale and markedly depressed
despite treatment with an antidepressant drug. He was now suffering
from severe constant bilateral abdominal and episodic back pain that
was not relieved by his current treatment. He was clearly approaching
the end of his life (the terminal stage of a terminal illness) but his death
was not necessarily imminent.

This man was commenced on continuous treatment with
morphine and maxolon (an anti-emetic) by injection, and a full range
of laboratory tests was ordered. It was decided that he would not be
resuscitated if his heart stopped (this was quite reasonable, but there was
no indication as to whether this was discussed with him or his wife),
and questions concerning further investigation of his spine by specialised
X-rays, further radiation or rehabilitation were all mooted. On 7 July
he was given a blood transfusion for his anaemia. On 8 July he was
'distressed, in abdominal pain, and unable to talk'.

The consultant saw him on 9 July and decided that further
investigation of clinical problems was irrelevant and that sedation be
continued. Later that day, the record indicates he had 'continued deterioration', was 'not verbalising, distressed by any movement' and had a
depressed 'conscious state'. These features were further discussed with
the consultant, and with the man's wife, and the decision was taken 'for
palliative care, analgesia, keep comfortable, cease oral medications'. This
was an eminently reasonable decision to cease treatment except for that
designed for comfort, and to concentrate on relief of suffering.

The nursing notes are more revealing of the exact state of affairs
over the next six days and the significant entries are as follows:

7/7/94—2100 hrs—complaining of back pain, requiring breakthrough doses of morphine mixture … feeling miserable
tonight, just wanting to go to sleep

8/7/94—1435 hrs—patient has had severe pain for the entire shift.
Several doses of subcutaneous morphine and morphine mixture given with moderate result … patient is also constipated
but cannot sit on pan because of excruciating pain in the back

2120 hrs—Subcutaneous morphine and midazolam infusion
commenced

9/7/94—1440 hrs—pain relief adequate when still, however pain
present when rolled

2000 hrs—pain and agitation … pain control inadequate this p.m.
both at rest and severe on movement morphine 200 mg,
lorezepam [sedative] 1mg given for agitation

10/7/94—0400 hrs—pain fairly controlled overnight except
when turning

1410 hrs—patient drowsy but rousable to verbal stimuli mouth
very dry

2055 hrs—morphine 300 mg, midazolam 2.5 mg

11/7/94—0400 hrs—still is in pain when turned

2100 hrs—becomes distressed when position is changed

12/7/94—0505 hrs—patient was very distressed and screaming
at beginning of shift

1400 hrs—patient still remains quite distressed when moving him

2100 hrs—morphine 400 mg, midazolam 5 mg still complains of
pain on movement

13/7/94—0510 hrs—patient has slept through the night

14/7/94 respiratory rate has slowed patient unresponsive

15/7/94 patient died.

The midazolam referred to is a short-acting sedative drug, which was
being infused to keep him asleep. It is obvious that this man's very severe

pain on movement could not be controlled by continuous morphine alone, even in large doses.

This situation was clearly similar to that of Betty in chapter 1, but the treatment, twenty years later, was very different. It was not, however, until the dose of morphine and sedative rendered the man deeply unconscious, having been gradually increased over five days during which he remained in distress, that the pain was relieved—at this level, it also depressed his breathing to lethal levels.

As was the custom in public hospitals at that time, an autopsy was performed and this revealed there was considerable spread of prostate cancer into the skeleton, but no evidence of any visceral spread (that is, into major organs such as heart, lungs, liver, kidneys or brain), and gross constipation was also present. It is clear from this post-mortem report the patient had not died from extensive spread of cancer into areas of the body that would cause serious organ dysfunction. This is not uncommon with prostate cancer, which is why dying is so slow and painful in this disease. The post-mortem and the clinical record clearly indicate the death was due to respiratory depression caused by the medication used for palliation and not specifically due to the cancer. No report of the death was made to the coroner, presumably because it was considered to be 'natural'.

I was astonished, to put it mildly, to read this medical record for many reasons. First, the death summary suggested that, after some minor problems, this man's death was a relatively comfortable and benign process. Such a conclusion is a mockery of the truth. The nursing record clearly indicates that he had continuing pain of varying, but often severe, degree from his admission on 5 July through to 13 July despite continuous medication and repeated adjustments to his medication. His palliative care did not provide maximum relief of his suffering or 'good symptom control' until the last forty-eight hours of his admission, when he was finally rendered unconscious until he died. Had I read the publication by Ivan Lichter and Esther Hunt entitled *The Last 48 Hours* I would not have been surprised. It included the following paragraph:

'The patient died peacefully at 0630 hours'. This is a report made by a nurse attending a patient's death. The wording is almost invariably the same—'the patient died peacefully'. Though the entry accurately describes the dying and the period immediately prior to death, there are times when these words do not tell the whole story. Unless it is taken in conjunction with a review of the comfort of the patient in the days preceding death, it may lead to an acceptance that all has been well. The peaceful death should not obscure the problems that sometimes arise in the last period of a terminal illness. At this time additional measures may be needed to ensure the patient's comfort. Patients certainly do die peacefully, but the final days may be difficult for the patient, the family and the carers.[2]

Second, the patient had clearly received treatment that had resulted in the hastening of his death. A person with even extensive bony metastatic disease causing paraplegia is not in a condition where one would expect a rapid progression to death, and a person can remain in this condition, such as Betty, for a significant period of time. Death usually occurs when major organs (such as heart, lungs, liver, kidneys or brain) are seriously affected and serious metabolic problems thereby ensue. Except for anaemia, this patient had no serious metabolic problems. The clinical notes indicate that he progressed to unconsciousness with depressed breathing, indicating that respiratory depression was his mode of death, and that this was clearly due to his treatment. In addition, he had an inadequate fluid intake to sustain adequate hydration (due to him being rendered drowsy or unconscious) and dehydration would have also contributed to his death. Despite this, no report of his death was made to the coroner.

The *Coroners Act 1985* (Vic) states that a death is reportable if it is 'unnatural', or if it occurs during an anaesthetic. This man's death, being clearly due to the drug medication that he received, could hardly be described as natural, and since the drugs used had deliberately induced coma, it could be argued that this was due to an anaesthetic process. In my view, on both of these grounds, his death should have been reported to the coroner for assessment. Third, there is no indication in the record that the use of this treatment was discussed with the patient, although it was with his wife. I accept that it might have been impossible to discuss it with the patient because of his altered mental state due to medication, but there is little if any evidence of an open, clear communication between the patient and the relative(s) concerning this man's predicament and a discussion of the options that were available.

To me, this death raised three essential concerns. First was the apparent lack of detailed discussion to find out the patient's wishes, there being no record that he or his wife had requested this treatment. I have no doubt that his wife would have been grateful that his suffering had been shortened, but she, and he, might have wished for maximum relief of his pain at the outset rather than this stuttering approach to that state. I accept that he may have been unable to take part in such discussions, but nevertheless this represents hastening of his death without his specific, or to use the word in the Dutch definition of euthanasia, explicit request. Second, despite the institution of palliative care which effectively led to this man's hastened death, inadequate control of symptoms was the case throughout the major part of his admission. Third, although his death clearly had been hastened by medical treatment, his death was not reported to the coroner.

Of course, I was aware that the use of high doses of morphine to ease death was a very old medical practice, surely as old as analgesics themselves, but here was, to me, a new practice—the deliberate and continuous use of sedatives to render a patient, whose death was not imminent, unconscious without hydration or the usual care of the airway of an unconscious patient, and maintaining that process until death. The process could be foreseen to probably or certainly hasten death, and yet no measures were taken to prevent death.

A number of questions needed answers. Why was there no apparent discussion with the patient? Why did it take so long to achieve adequate symptom control when the nursing record clearly indicated that he had persistent continuing severe pain? Was this a common palliative care practice? If it was, was it also common practice not to report such deaths to the coroner, in clear breach of the statute? I determined to find out more about this type of palliative care practice and the coroner's attitude towards it.

I began to read the refereed palliative care journals, and found a wealth of information regarding the efficiency of palliative care when critically assessed by both experts and the recipients of that care and their relatives. References to the use of sedation with midazolam first appeared in 1988 and increased in frequency to the present time. Emile de Sousa and Bridget Jepson reported:

> Of 157 patients who died at this hospice between July and October, 1987, 99 (65.6%) received subcutaneous infusions of diamorphine (heroin) in the terminal phase of their disease ... Several such patients require sedation ... We found Midazolam in combination with Diamorphine (and when necessary Hyoscine) to be an effective sedative for continuous subcutaneous infusion administration.[3]

In 1990, an Italian group writing in *Palliative Care* reported:

> The lack of control of physical suffering among cancer patients in the last days or hours of life is a common problem, but is rarely discussed in an open fashion ... 52.5% of terminal cancer patients treated at home by palliative care teams had physical symptoms unendurable to the patient and controllable only by sedation-inducing sleep on average two days before death. The most common symptoms included breathlessness (50%), pain (50%), delirium (20%) and vomiting (8%). More than 50% of these patients die with physical suffering that is controllable only by means of sedation.[4]

In 1990, Bottomly and Hanks recommended a subcutaneous midazolam infusion for terminal restlessness and agitation, and stated:

> Restlessness and agitation are common problems in advanced cancer patients in the final days of life. Restlessness and agitation in a patient who is dying may cause considerable distress, not only to the patient, but also to the family, and active intervention is indicated.[5]

With refreshing honesty (compared to many other palliative care experts) they said, 'Respiratory depression is more likely when Midazolam is used together with opioid analgesics'.

This approach was rapidly accepted by Australian hospices, with Burke and colleagues writing in 1991 in the *Medical Journal of Australia* that midazolam was used for terminal 'restlessness' in eighty-six patients during a 10-month period:

> Initially the use of the drug was infrequent. Fourteen patients received the drug in the first four months; in the following six months, the drug was used in 72 patients.
>
> Midazolam was found to be an effective drug in every case except one. It provided a readily available means of controlling symptoms and overcoming patient distress where no feasible alternative existed previously.
>
> During the last six months, almost 20% of inpatients received Midazolam, compared with 2% of home care patients.[6]

One wonders how bad were deaths before the introduction of sedation. It would be intriguing to know the incidence of terminal sedation in home-care patients in 2007.

Professor R G Twycross, the doyen of British palliative care experts, writing in the *Oxford Textbook of Palliative Medicine* (1993), advised deep sedation for the management of terminal anguish. He commented that nothing short of deep unconsciousness could provide relief and that inadequate sedation makes matters worse.

NI Cherny and his co-workers, in a paper entitled 'The Treatment of Suffering when Patients Request Elective Death', wrote:

> For some patients with advanced disease, adequate relief of physical symptoms may only be achieved at the cost of profound sedation. The incidence of this situation is controversial and has been variably estimated at between 5% and 52%.
>
> Refractory delirium may be associated with severe agitation, refractory depression, anxiety or existential distress. Persistent patient distress of this kind places great stress upon the resources of family, friends and professional health care providers. Indeed the combination of distress, fatigue and perceived therapeutic destitution may be such that death is seen as the preferred option.[7]

Further expert Australian comment came from Professor Michael Ashby of Monash University, who summed up the situation in clear fashion in 1995:

> Heavy sedation may be used to induce a state of impaired consciousness to control so-called terminal restlessness, or when symptoms and suffering cannot be controlled by other palliative treatments.
>
> This practice has been termed 'pharmacological oblivion'; the Canadian Senate calls it 'total sedation' or the 'practice of rendering a person totally unconscious through the administration of drugs without potentially shortening life'. Such treatment is argued to be within accepted palliative care practice, as the death is not intended, and the doctrine of double effect applies, although it is surely impossible to state that such treatment does not have the potential to shorten life.
>
> It is sometimes argued that intentional shortening of life may be justified if requested by a terminally ill patient, and that

so-called 'pharmacological oblivion' (using sedation to make
a person drowsy or unconscious while they are dying) is merely
a rationalisation of what the medical practitioner is really doing.[8]

Some clarification of this possibility came from Dr Alan Fleischman:
'terminal sedation is justified to alleviate pain and suffering whilst
acknowledging that death is not only a risk but a likelihood'.[9]

It required more reading to realise that in the majority of circumstances
where deep sedation was used there was no provision of food and fluids,
no specific care of the airway that is usually the case in unconscious
patients, and no monitoring of vital signs. In other words, it is accepted
that the patient will die and that such measures are not provided as they
would provide no benefit and simply prolong the dying process.

It was very clear that this practice of 'pharmacological oblivion'
(now more commonly called 'terminal sedation', which sounds more
benign, but even this description causes some in palliative care much
angst) was well established in palliative care practice, was becoming
increasingly common, and was filling a very important role in relieving terminal suffering. It certainly was not often discussed, as Ventafridda
said, in an open fashion (I had discovered its use only by accident), and
there was only a grudging admission it could hasten death. It was, however, clearly a palliative act and one that seemed clinically necessary and
humane. On the other hand, 'voluntary euthanasia' was a medical intervention that hastened the death of terminally ill patients in order to
relieve their suffering and such action was widely believed to be criminal. Here was a practice, widely accepted in palliative care, which hastened the death of some terminally ill patients in order to relieve their
suffering, but which was apparently not criminal and appeared to be
hidden from the coroner. Two palliative practices—one legal, the other
considered illegal!

I wrote to the coroner in October 1995 seeking his advice as to
whether a death due to terminal sedation was a reportable death, thus

requiring the scrutiny of the coronial process. In reply, he sent me a copy of the *Coroners Act 1985* (Vic), and drew my attention to Section 3 (e–g), but did not specifically answer my question. He also sent a copy of my letter to the Attorney-General. The relevant section states a 'reportable death' means:

> a death (e) that appears to have been unexpected, unnatural, or violent or to have resulted, directly or indirectly, from an accident or injury; or (f) that occurs during an anaesthetic; or (g) that occurs as a result of an anaesthetic and is not due to natural causes.

The key words are 'unnatural' and 'anaesthetic', but they are not defined by the Act. An anaesthetic is a deliberate process where a patient may be rendered unconscious for therapeutic purposes (the prevention or relief of pain), and normally the person's life is stringently protected in anticipation of uneventful recovery. Terminal sedation is a deliberate process where a patient is rendered unconscious for therapeutic purposes, but their life is not protected since death rather than an uneventful recovery is not only anticipated but certain (and perhaps welcome!).

An unnatural death is presumably the antithesis of a natural death, a complex concept in this age when few deaths occur in the absence of medical intervention. It would be generally accepted that a natural death is one due to old age or disease, and not caused by human intervention, such as dying during one's sleep. It is reasonable to suppose that the coroner exists to study death due to human intervention to ensure that it is not criminal or avoidable. In my view, terminal sedation, by causing respiratory depression, by causing dehydration, by failing to adequately protect the airway of an unconscious patient leading to potentially fatal pulmonary complications, is an intervention that can cause an unnatural death. The fact that there is a fatal disease process in train at the same time, which is a competing cause of death, obscures the issue as to whether the death is natural or unnatural. Without some definition or guidance, the medical practitioner is in a dilemma as to what is reportable and what is not. This was the advice that I sought from the coroner, but which he would not provide.

The Attorney-General replied (28 November 1995), stating that 'Your inquiry raises a matter of public importance' and that she would seek legal advice upon it. The Attorney-General's further letter of 17 January 1996 advised that

> a death occurring during or as a result of the process of pharma-cological oblivion itself may qualify as a 'reportable death' ... Even if a death is from natural causes, I am advised that the death would be 'reportable' if it occurred during an anaesthetic [and] instances may occur where a doctor is unable to determine the cause of death of a person who has died during or as a result of the process of pharmacological oblivion itself. I am advised that in those instances the doctor is required to report the death.

Clearly, this advice indicated that at least some deaths occurring in palliative care due to pharmacological oblivion should be reported to the coroner but it seemed to me that this was not occurring. Nobody seemed to mind that the deaths of some terminally ill patients were being hastened, provided it was done slowly and no one complained.

I clearly had no involvement in this man's death. I do not know the intentions of those providing his care except the obvious intention to provide palliation. Jessica Corner's statement introducing this chapter indicates that multiple intentions commonly may be present in this situation—the intention both to palliate suffering and to hasten death—and to my mind this is totally reasonable, and to be expected. But to date terminal sedation continues behind closed doors.

10

RESPECTING CHOICE

*'Making someone die in a way others approve, but he believes a
horrifying contradiction of his life, is a devastating,
odious form of tyranny.'*[1]
Professor Ronald Dworkin, Professor of Law, New York University

During 1996, I received a telephone call from a very distressed man
concerning his 85-year-old father Harold, who had been admitted
to a major teaching hospital with a brain stem stroke. This form of stroke
affects a particularly important part of the brain and has devastating effects.
The slender narrow area emerging from the base of the brain which
carries the nerve tracts from the brain to the spinal cord is destroyed.
Typically, such a situation involves total paralysis except for the ability to
move the eyes. There is total inability to speak or swallow, whilst still being
able to see and hear. Basic heart and breathing functions are preserved.
Even more terrifying, the cognitive functions of the brain are usually not
impaired. One can think, but there is absolutely no way in which thoughts
can be expressed. There is rarely if ever any likelihood of any recovery
from this state. It has been described, understandably, as a 'locked-in' state.

Harold's treating neurologists had inserted a PEG feeding tube (a tube placed through the abdominal wall into the stomach) to allow feeding and hydration, since Harold could not swallow. With continued feeding via this means, he could remain alive for months or years. Even the extreme anti-euthanasia advocate Professor Norelle Lickiss has stated that if she ever had the misfortune to have such a stroke she would not want her life prolonged by a feeding tube.

This was the dilemma faced by Harold and his family, and it was exactly such a dilemma that Harold had been at pains to avoid. He had been a member of the Voluntary Euthanasia Society of Victoria for some years, and had followed that Society's advice to appoint an agent (medical enduring power of attorney) to make medical decisions if he ever became incompetent to do so. That had now occurred and his son, as his agent, was certain that his father would not wish to be kept alive in these circumstances by tube feeding. He was seeking my advice in order to have the tube feeding ceased.

Whenever a person has a major stroke, the immediate effects can appear devastating, but significant (although usually incomplete) recovery can occur with time and medical support. Recovery is very unlikely after a brain stem stroke, but a period of support is not unreasonable, particularly in young patients. The fascinating book *The Diving-Bell and the Butterfly*[2] describes the story of a 42-year-old survivor of such a stroke. Despite his relatively young age, he had made no recovery from his original situation. Nevertheless, he wrote his book via an amanuensis using merely the remaining movement of his left eyelid. A young person might want to explore such an opportunity but it is unlikely in an 85-year-old, and it was not what Harold wanted—he had already made that abundantly clear to his son, his legally appointed agent. The initial decision to place the tube was not seriously opposed as it had been advised by experienced neurologists on the basis that some recovery might be possible, but after ten days with no such occurrence, the futility of the situation was becoming apparent to the family. They asked for the tube to be removed but their request was deflected.

The Victorian *Medical Treatment Act* was passed in 1988 following the recommendations of an all-party Parliamentary Committee of Inquiry into Dying with Dignity. Many countries have similar legislation. It confirmed in the statute law the existing common law right for any competent person to refuse any medical treatment. This excluded palliative care, defined as 'the reasonable provision of food and water', and 'provision of reasonable medical procedures for the relief of pain, suffering and discomfort'. This Act, in its preamble, states:

> The Parliament recognizes that it is desirable—
> (a) to give protection to the patient's right to refuse unwanted medical treatment;
> (b) to give protection to medical practitioners who act in good faith in accordance with a patient's express wishes;
> (c) to recognize the difficult circumstances that face medical practitioners in advising and providing guidance in relation to treatment options; ...
> (f) to ensure that dying patients receive maximum relief of pain and suffering.

The Act also created the right to appoint an agent to make medical decisions if one became unable to make one's own decisions (incompetent). Unfortunately, like much legislation, it is little known or understood by the public, although it should be well known to the medical profession. However, research carried out by Melbourne's Monash University investigators in 2001 revealed that only 7 per cent of doctors had a thorough understanding of this Act and 44 per cent had a totally inadequate knowledge of it.[3]

I advised Harold's son of his father's rights under the Act, transferred to him as his agent. I believed he had the right to ask for the tube feeding to be ceased and for his father to be provided with whatever palliation was necessary to keep him comfortable following cessation of hydration. The original decision to place the tube was reasonable, in order to allow for any possible recovery, but when this failed to occur, it was surely unreasonable to persist. Should the consequences of such an initial decision to treat be irrevocable? I did not think so. His treating doctors, however, would still not comply with the son's request, and so I arranged a meeting with Harold's family—wife, son and two daughters—at his home to discuss the matter.

At the family meeting, it was completely obvious that every member of the family was in no doubt what Harold's view of the situation would have been if he could have expressed it—don't continue to feed me to keep me alive in this situation; let me die with some dignity. Even if Harold's son did not have medical enduring power of attorney I believed that, if the whole family was of one mind, the tube could be removed and no further fluids given (though they should still be offered). The position was even stronger having appointed an enduring medical power of attorney to legally make decisions if Harold became unable to do so.

Whilst it would be possible to arrange for tube feeding to cease, should this husband and father have to then die of dehydration, while still being cognitively aware? I did not think that was acceptable, and told the family that I believed that Harold could be kept sedated to prevent any distressing effects from lack of fluids on the basis of providing maximum relief of pain and suffering (as specified in the *Medical Treatment Act 1988*), even if such action hastened his inevitable death. I explained this carefully to the family, whilst also pointing out that this aspect of the Act had not been tested in the courts and that, strictly speaking, in view of my correspondence with the coroner, I should probably report the anticipated death to the coroner. Harold's wife, who was eighty-seven, was extremely fearful of the effects on her of such a report, and so I agreed that it would not be done.

After very careful and detailed discussion, it was agreed that Harold's son would request that his father be transferred to my hospital, where I would accede to his request to cease feeding via the PEG tube and keep him completely comfortable with sedation. This duly occurred, and after completing the appropriate legally binding Refusal of Treatment certificate, the feeding was ceased and after five days of sedation Harold died peacefully, having spent his last three days in a coma.

Clearly this was a new level of assistance in dying for me. It was based on my careful reading of the *Medical Treatment Act 1988* (Vic). It seemed quite clear to me that the Act would allow a legally appointed agent to refuse medical treatment, in this case artificial hydration and nutrition, with the secondary provision of sedation to palliate any suffering that occurred due to that withdrawal of treatment. I had intended in this matter to conform to the law. I had studied the Act and sought advice from the highest relevant legal officers. Nevertheless, it took me into a complex legal and ethical arena, which was to test me severely for more than a decade.

There is virtually no doubt that world-wide expert medical opinion would agree that artificial feeding of any kind (by intravenous or gastric tube access) is medical treatment and can be refused by a competent patient. In 1992, it was the opinion of the Council of Judicial and Ethical Affairs of the American Medical Association that life-prolonging medical treatment included medication and artificially supplied respiration, nutrition or hydration.[4] The eminent neurologist JL Bernat, writing in *Ethical Issues in Neurology*, stated that for incompetent patients without hope of recovery, 'hydration and nutrition are provided, encouraged and assisted orally, but they are not administered parenterally or via a feeding tube unless they improve the patient's comfort or are explicitly ordered by a legally authorised surrogate'.[5] He also said it may be rational for a patient to escape a life of intractable suffering, rather than to continue living in a 'locked-in state'.[6] The United States Supreme Court Justice Sandra Day O'Connor stated in *Cruzan v. Director* that 'artificial feeding cannot readily be distinguished from other forms of medical treatment ... Accordingly the liberty guaranteed by the Due Process Clause must protect, if it protect anything, an individual's deeply personal decision to reject medical treatment including the artificial delivery of food and water'.[7]

The *Medical Treatment Act*, in the preamble quoted earlier, leads to a reasonable expectation, and a legal right, that the rights of a competent person should be transferred to their agent if that person should become incompetent. However, it was possible at that time for some doctors to argue that the refusal of artificial hydration was an uncertain right under the Act, and that such hydration might be considered palliative care. It could be argued that the provision of fluids could be for the comfort of the patient, despite the fact that any such discomfort can be readily relieved by analgesics and sedatives. How could I know whether Harold had any suffering since he could not communicate? I could not but think for a moment of his indescribable distress if he had suffering and could not say so or indicate it in any way.

Undoubtedly I assisted in hastening Harold's death by agreeing to his agent's request for withdrawal of artificial hydration and by providing sedation to palliate any suffering thus created. My intention was to respect his autonomy and legal right to refuse unwanted treatment, and the sedation was in response to his right to maximal relief of pain and suffering.

Over the past eleven years I have been involved in a number of cases where the right of a person to refuse a feeding tube, or to have one removed, has arisen. In early 2002, a 92-year-old woman was admitted to a major Melbourne teaching hospital with a severe stroke, and despite the objections of her legally appointed agent, a naso-gastric tube was inserted. Despite approaches by her agent to the highest hospital authorities, the Health Services Commissioner and the Public Advocate, the tube remained, the hospital obtaining legal opinion that it was obliged to provide reasonable food and fluids, interpreted as including tube feeding. She died seven months later in a nursing home. This was an outcome that she profoundly wished to avoid, and had actually taken steps to do so.

This woman's fate is an example of Ivan Illich's 'medicalisation of death'.[8] At ninety-two, her severe stroke was clearly a terminal or pre-terminal event, yet her doctors insisted on providing treatment that would prolong her life in a futile and unwanted manner.

PEG feeding was introduced into medicine only in 1979, but by 1999 it was estimated that 34 per cent of severely demented nursing home patients in Boston had PEG feeding tubes. By 2005 it was estimated that 225 000 such tubes were in place in the United States in patients over sixty-five.[9] Another American study found that 47 per cent of a group of elderly cancer and dementia patients received invasive non-palliative treatments during their final few days. Of patients with dementia, 51 per cent received tube feeding and all still had the feeding tube in place at death![10] This simply illustrates that if a life-preserving treatment is available, then doctors are very likely to use it, despite the context. No matter that the treatment is likely to be futile and simply prolong dying. A doctor may gain respect by being brutally honest and pointing out such futility, but the default medical position is always to treat, based on fear of prosecution for negligence, or perhaps alleged intention to hasten death. Towards the end of his life Illich wrote, 'While doctors concentrated on the fight against death, the patient became a residual object, then a technological construct. Today, one asks: is there still an autonomous self capable of the act of dying?'[11]

The answer is yes, but only if one is prepared and informed. This is why it is essential that everybody appoint a medical enduring power of attorney, and create an advance directive to defeat that default decision.

An advance directive is a witnessed document that sets out, in clear terms, what treatment a person does or does not want if they are unable to express their wishes in relation to some future event. It should be designed to refuse treatment only if a catastrophic event occurs in which recovery is highly unlikely and treatment will only prolong life in a futile manner. Such documents are of value to both patients and their doctors. Carefully developed and precise advance directives are available from Dying With Dignity Victoria. Unfortunately, the *Medical Treatment Act* recognises refusal of treatment for only 'a current condition', and does not recognise the concept of an advance directive. However, without legal certainty doctors are reluctant to act to protect their patient's autonomy. Mukesh Haikerwal (AMA Federal president at the time) commented:

> Doctors should take notice of advance directives—written statements which set out a patient's treatment preferences—but the problem is getting doctors to recognize their legal status. We are not far enough along the path in this area for doctors to accept these are legal directions that must be adhered [to].[12]

Despite the clear intentions of the *Medical Treatment Act 1988* (Vic) to protect the right of patients to refuse treatment and to receive maximum relief of pain and suffering, there are doctors who deliberately prevent such outcomes. Sometimes this is because of unforgivable lack of knowledge, sometimes because of unreasonable fear of the law, and sometimes because of their moral point of view. Doctors should recognise, however, that they are not moral arbiters. Dr Brian Pollard, an anaesthetist, Catholic medical ethicist and opponent of euthanasia, wrote about 'withdrawing life-sustaining treatment from severely brain-damaged persons'. He said:

> Some ethicists regard the removal of a feeding tube from patients in a persistent vegetative state as direct killing. Since food is necessary to the continuation of life, they argue that the denial of nutrition is a form of murder. They are inconsistent, however, if they permit the removal of a ventilator, since air is as necessary to life as food. Yet other ethicists advance a concept of human life which embraces philosophical and theological concepts, as well as physiological. They would support the removal of tube feeding in these patients, provided the criteria could be objectively confirmed. They argue that human life does not consist alone of functioning physiology. Physiology serves the higher purposes

of life, such as thinking, experiencing emotions, forming human relationships and being able to pursue, at least at some minimal level, a spiritual component of life. If it can be shown in an individual that these capacities have been permanently lost, life in its human fullness is already lacking. This position is not based on an assessment of the quality of life, but on the absence of complete life as they conceive it.[13]

Sophistry aside, this expounds a liberal Catholic position, accepted by many except the ultra-conservative believers in the sanctity of life under any circumstances (such as Right to Life, the highly conservative Catholic-based Australian pro-life group). Conservative Catholic bioethicists believe that there is a basic level of care for health and life that patients are obliged to accept, or carers to provide. Such a liberal position as Pollard's was not accepted by the late Pope John Paul II, who told the World Federation of Catholic Medical Associations and the Pontifical Academy for Life, in 2004, that 'If this [withdrawal of food and fluids] is knowingly and deliberately carried out, this would result in a true euthanasia by omission' and that the provision of food and water by artificial means to a person in a permanently vegetative state was 'morally obligatory'. This caused consternation among many Catholic doctors.

By 2002, some fourteen years after the *Medical Treatment Act 1988* (Vic) was passed, the question of refusal of, or withdrawal of, feeding tubes in incompetent patients was still unresolved. Apart from the influence of factors mentioned above, there was lack of clarity in the Act as to whether artificial feeding was palliative care or medical treatment.

In June 2002, I was contacted by a man whose 67-year-old wife (BWV), suffering from profound dementia, had been fed via a PEG (stomach) tube for seven years and was now in a permanent vegetative state in a nursing home. I visited her and found that she was bed-bound, lying in a permanently contracted foetal position, completely unable to interact with her environment, biologically but not biographically alive. However, to my observation, she had a primal ability to demon-strate distress. Her husband had been trying for two years to have the tube feeding stopped without success, the doctor and the nursing home stating that the law did not allow them to remove the tube.

BWV had not appointed her husband as her legally appointed agent, but even if he were, the law was still obscure to her doctor, who was not prepared to respect the request. I advised him to make an appli-cation to the Victorian Civil and Administrative Tribunal (VCAT) to appoint a guardian, who could legally make the decision to cease tube feeding. Eventually, this application was successful and the Public Advocate was so appointed. It was still possible that the doctor could refuse the request on the grounds that tube feeding was palliative care.

In order to put this matter beyond dispute, the Public Advocate took the matter to the Supreme Court of Victoria for a declaration. Mr Justice Morris confirmed VCAT's decision; more importantly, he declared that artificial feeding was a medical treatment.[14] BWV died twenty-one days after tube feeding was ceased, but nine months after the application to VCAT was made, and three years after the first request was made.

In relation to this particular case, Professor Michael Ashby made this beguiling statement about artificial feeding for dying patients: 'There's a myth about that people who are dying of some form of fatal process or illness, unless they're artificially fed, they suffer the ill-effects of starvation. We see no evidence of that.'[15] It is beguiling because it is partially correct, but thereby deceptive. First, the failure to provide artificial feeding creates lack of both food and fluids, but the principal suffering of such patients is of dehydration, not starvation. Thirst is a much more powerful distress than hunger. It is true that if patients are very close to death, they will show no desire for food or fluids, as though their body has shut down completely in its needs. Moreover, if the patient is comatose, due to disease or sedation, then no distress will be evident. But patients who are fully conscious and fully hydrated and not close to death, although having an ultimately fatal illness, can be expected to experience as much suffering as you or I if we were deprived of food and fluids.

Palliative care makes much of good patient care with mouth toilets (keeping the mouth and lips moist), but can this palliate the existential distress of conscious persons whose only option is to dehydrate themselves to death? And how does one know if there is distress when depriving a patient in a conscious, but uncommunicative, state of fluids when the patient may be quite incapable of expressing such distress? Such is the case for a person in a 'locked-in state' like Harold, or persistent vegetative state like BWV. Clearly, it is the context that matters.

A different view from Ashby's was expressed by Dr Philip Howard in a letter to *The [London] Times* in which he said, 'Withdrawal of fluids will cause the patient to die from dehydration, which is distressing to the patient, to the carers, and to relatives. It is disingenuous and inhumane to suggest to the contrary'.[16]

Howard was actually arguing against withdrawing fluids, but his statement is just as powerful as support for adequate sedation when fluids are withdrawn. In my opinion, if there is the slightest chance that a patient might suffer from the withdrawal of food and fluids, then sufficient sedation to eliminate that suffering should be offered and provided unless the patient, or their agent, refuses it.

VCAT is a legal tribunal comprising senior legal and judicial members. Both they and Mr Justice Morris drew heavily on the precedent set by the Law Lords in the similar Bland case in Britain in 1993. The Law Lords wrote of that case:

> it is not about euthanasia, if by that is meant the taking of positive action to cause death [yet another definition of euthanasia]. It is not about putting down the old and the infirm, the mentally defective or the physically imperfect [not that such a suggestion has ever been made in the name of medically assisted dying] the issue is whether artificial feeding ... may lawfully be withheld from ... [a] patient [in this condition who has] no hope of recovery

when it is known that if that is done the patient will shortly thereafter die.[17]

VCAT accepted the submission of the Public Advocate that 'the provision of food and water cannot be said to be reasonable when it is provided to a person who is dying, not for the primary purpose of palliation, but with the aim of deferring or suspending the process of dying'.[18] The Law Lords also said, 'We emphasise this point especially: the question is never whether the patient's life is worthwhile but whether the treatment is worthwhile'.[19]

VCAT's judgment had to be based on legal principle and, if possible, precedent. Thus its decision that the tube feeding was medical, not palliative, treatment, that it was unreasonable provision of food and fluids, that it was not worthwhile (that is, futile), and that it was not euthanasia, were legal judgments supported by sound medical opinion. The questions they asked were necessarily legal questions, but, as such, lack a human dimension. That was provided by the presentation of the family who clearly argued that their loved one 'had no quality of life', that although she was incompetent she was suffering, and that for those reasons she should be allowed to die. The family saw the problem in a completely different context from the court.

Further, the Tribunal, while acknowledging that 'the patient will shortly die thereafter', did not address the nature of the dying—the questions 'how will she die and how will we deal with it?' were not addressed. Perhaps they were right not to do so, as this is a medical question, but it is a medical question that is charged with legal issues. If the tube feeding is ceased, the person will die of dehydration. Since that process starts from a position of full hydration, it will usually take between seven and fourteen days. BWV was described as being in a vegetative state, so she could not indicate if she had any suffering or ask for any palliation. However, she was, in my opinion, not totally insensate. Surely, therefore, there could not be allowed even the slightest chance that she could suffer in any way as that legally ordained but macabre process unfolded. Sophisticated neurological studies have revealed that a residual pain-related cerebral network remained active in some persistant vegetative state (PVS) patients.[20] BWV should have been palliated by being kept asleep from the time the feeding ceased until she died. It was reported that she received 'palliative care' but of what kind is unknown.

Again, a doctor sees this matter in a completely different context from the court. As a doctor I would ask the court how is it possible to impose a slow death by dehydration on a human being? It would be illegal for a domestic animal, or for any animal. If the law did not condone certain hastening of death by deliberate sedation to relieve suffering, could it not at least condone the certain relief of suffering by deliberate sedation that might hasten death?

Even with sedation, this is an awful process for the relatives, nurses and doctors; a time of stress and futility. Since the Tribunal cited futility as a reason for ceasing the tube feeding, might it not have addressed the futility and suffering of the consequences of such an action? Clearly such a process of palliation, by prolonged sedation, is not a good process. Is there not a better palliative process?

This BWV decision was concerned with the following values:

- the autonomy (via surrogate expression) of BWV and her best interests (legal and ethical values)
- futility of treatment and the necessity to relieve suffering (medical and human values)
- quality of life and relief of suffering (human values). These were certainly the reasons expressed by the family, even if ignored by the court.

Both VCAT and the Supreme Court accepted that this was a genuine request by the patient's family (her surrogate decision makers), who were fully informed of the consequences of withdrawal of tube feeding. The cessation of tube feeding, authorised by the court, was a deliberate act that hastened death. It was not explicitly requested by BWV, but was by her family as her surrogates. This was the intention of BWV, as expressed by her family, in order to end her suffering. Apart from the lack of dignity in dying by dehydration, these conditions fulfil my definition of euthanasia, but not the rather pitiful definition of the Law Lords.

Justice Morris did not comment on the question of euthanasia, confining himself to the legal question of whether tube feeding was medical treatment or palliative care. He did, however, refer to 'sanctity of life', which was raised frequently by the counsel for Right to Life and the Catholic Church. Their view of sanctity was based on concepts of holiness, pureness, sacredness and dedication of life to God. Justice Morris, presiding over a secular court, indicated that this principle is better referred to as 'the inviolability of life'. He referred, as did VCAT, to the statement of Lord Hoffman in the House of Lords' decision in the Bland case (a very similar situation to BWV).

> But the sanctity of life is only one of a cluster of ethical principles which we apply to decisions about how we live. Another is respect for the individual human being and in particular for his right to choose how he should live his own life. We call this individual autonomy or the right to self-determination. And another principle, closely connected, is respect for the dignity of the individual human being: our belief that quite irrespective of what the person concerned may think about it, it is wrong for someone to be humiliated or treated without respect for his value as a person.
>
> I do not suggest that the position which English law has taken is the only morally correct position. Some might think that in cases of life and death, the law should be more paternalistic even to adults. The point to be emphasized is that there is no morally correct solution which can be deduced from a single ethical principle like the sanctity of life or the right to self-determination.

There must be an accommodation between principles, both of which seem rational and good but which have come into conflict with each other.[21]

Justice Morris agreed with Lord Hoffman regarding the balance between these competing values, which revolves around the 'best interests' of the patient. In both Bland and BWV, autonomy trumped sanctity of life. Thankfully, Justice Morris's decision should protect many Victorians from unwanted prolongation of life in futile and undignified circumstances. It was a brave decision in controversial circumstances— it would have been an even better decision if he had reminded the court of the necessity for dying patients to receive maximal relief of pain and suffering.

A right to live does not include an obligation to do so, under any or every circumstance. It is surely true that we can waive such a right, and this is the basis of our autonomy in end-of-life decisions.

11

A DIFFICULT SITUATION

*'Patients request a hastened death not simply because of unrelieved
pain, but because of a wide variety of unrelieved symptoms, in
combination with loss of meaning, dignity and independence.'*[1]

Dr Timothy Quill

Doctors' attitudes to voluntary euthanasia are a matter of great vari-
ation and some bewilderment. Published surveys of the attitudes
and actions of Australian doctors indicate that from 1988 to the
present, 40–60 per cent (varying according to state) support a change
in the law in Australia along the Dutch lines.[2] There are in addition a
number of doctors who want to be able to provide physician–assisted
dying for their patients but do not want the law to change. They are
happy to work in an illegal, covert, but in their view ethical, way in
order to keep the legal system from being involved in any way with
their practice. Medicine and the law approach problems in a very
different way and, like oil and water, do not mix well. It is my feeling
that those doctors who favour the status quo are predominantly
general practitioners, who can treat patients in the security of their

patient's home in an environment of long-standing trust and open communication with their patient and family. One can understand their distaste at having to comply with a formal process of documentation and reporting, second opinions and scrutiny, and a perception and fear that the law will be intimately involved in every end-of-life matter. There is no doubt the legal arrangements in the Netherlands are more exacting and time consuming than the nonexistent rules of covert practice. These arrangements are prescribed entirely for the benefit of the patient, and to ensure that mistakes are not made. Ultimately, they also benefit doctors who, if they are practising ethically, are protected from prosecution, and are able to help their patients in the choice of the most suitable way of relieving their suffering. They can also have the support of colleagues, in what are often difficult decisions, in a way that covert practice does not allow.

Specialists, on the other hand, largely working in the very public environment of a hospital, find great difficulty in responding to legit-imate patient requests, and have either to wash their hands of the matter, or employ the quasi-legal method of increasing doses of morphine (and sometimes sedatives) in order to relieve suffering and hasten death. As a means of trying to achieve a hastened death, this often proves to be non-voluntary, and tends to be rather crude and undignified. Due to circumstances, it is one of the commonest means of hastening death, but one of the least autonomous, least dignified and least effective.

I always wonder about the attitude of a doctor who suggests their patient comes to see me about an end-of-life matter, but without a referral letter. Do they approve of voluntary euthanasia in principle, but are not prepared to be personally involved? Are they frightened of legal consequences or harm to their reputation such that they will not even put pen to paper to provide relevant background information? Or do they personally disapprove, but accept that the patient has a right to explore such an option if it is their choice?

Keith, a 71-year-old retired company director, had three doctors involved in his care when he made an appointment to see me—his general practitioner of ten years, a surgeon who had made his diagnosis and was directing his treatment, and a medical specialist who had been involved in a procedural matter. None of these made the appointment or provided a referral letter. Keith had a short history of abdominal discomfort, associated with dark urine and pale faeces. His jaundice had been confirmed by a blood test, all of which suggested that his bile ducts were blocked. The CT scan had revealed a large (4 cm) irregular mass in the head of his pancreas, consistent with a cancer. There was no evidence of spread of cancer beyond the pancreas, which was highly likely to be the site of an incurable cancer.

Such a diagnosis carries a grave prognosis. A pancreatic cancer is often a very 'silent' cancer, not producing any symptoms until it is large and usually already incurable. Although Keith's presumed cancer did not show any obvious evidence of spread, and was therefore technically curable, the statistical chances of cure would be less than 5 per cent, and the operation is one of the most major abdominal procedures, with significant morbidity and operative mortality. The diagnosis was not 100 per cent certain as there was no histological proof (microscopic evidence) of cancer, but there is virtually no other possible diagnosis that produces this set of clinical circumstances. Keith apparently took little time to make up his mind that he would not undergo surgery. He did accept his surgeon's offer of the placement of a tube, using a flexible telescope, to relieve the blockage to the secretion of bile from his liver and relieve his jaundice.

When I saw Keith in late 1998, his main complaints were of loss of appetite, nausea and an ache in the right upper abdomen. He had lost about 7 kilograms in weight. He was not in pain. His medications were replacement pancreatic enzymes and the antidepressant Prothiaden. He had been married for forty-three years and his wife accompanied him to the consultation and sat in on the discussion. They had no children. I was not surprised when he asked for my help in providing him with euthanasia. I explained that I was sympathetic to the idea that he should have control over his future, but that providing such control was not simple, and that I would need to obtain confirmatory medical information from his surgeon. I arranged to see him again in two weeks.

His surgeon provided me with the necessary clinical information and confirmed that Keith had refused curative surgery. On review, his symptoms were unchanged except that he had lost more weight and was sleeping poorly. His discomfort was controlled by Panadeine (a simple oral analgesic). Once again I indicated my support but felt that his symptoms were hardly such that he would find life intolerable at this point. My own father had had a similar cancer and he refused surgery to relieve his jaundice. My father had been able to carry on for some months, finding significant value in his declining life, meeting with old friends and saying goodbye. I tried to persuade Keith to pursue those things that had given him interest in life before his diagnosis, but he was resistant to any idea other than ending his life. His devoted wife, who accompanied him on every occasion but said very little, did not seem inclined to support me.

There was no doubt that Keith had an incurable cancer and would die from it, probably in a few months time. However, he did not at present have intolerable physical symptoms that would justify my assistance. His situation was not one that would have justified terminal sedation. He seemed obsessed with avoiding a slow decline and decay, and even now could find no pleasure in life. Such a state of anhedonia is a singular marker for depression, although he was taking an anti-depressant drug. Was I underestimating his psychological and existential distress, or was he truly depressed? A psychiatric second opinion would have been helpful, but at this point I did not know of a psychiatrist to whom I could turn in such a delicate matter.

I now knew about barbiturates as the best means of assisting people like Keith, but there were difficulties in their prescription. Those drugs had been largely superseded by safer sedatives. They were well known for their lethal potential, and if Keith used my prescription to end his life, a very uncomfortable spotlight might turn on me. I was struggling in my mind with the risks of such a prescription, particularly in view of my public comments on physician-assisted dying.

In addition, I had recently had a phone call from the local police about my involvement in a tragic death. I had been phoned by a man seeking my help to die who, in a limited conversation, seemed to have serious psychological problems. I had advised him to seek psychiatric help. He subsequently self-immolated in a public place. I was, at this stage, extremely—perhaps even unreasonably—anxious about the question of prescribing barbiturates, particularly for any patient with whom I did not have an established clinical relationship.

In the interval since I last saw Keith, he had been admitted to hospital with vomiting and fever and some increase in abdominal pain, almost certainly an episode of cholangitis (infection of the ducts of the liver), a consequence of the tube in his bile duct to relieve his jaundice. He was now on antibiotics. A further CT scan had shown that the mass had increased to 5 cm. He had noted some further weight loss, and pain around the right lower ribs was being relieved by increased use of Panadeine (now six per day). He was suffering from nausea and I prescribed an anti-emetic (Maxolon), indicating that it would be useful at a later date to prevent vomiting when he ended his life.

When I saw Keith one week later, his principal complaints were of aching in the liver area, which was not well relieved by two panadeine tablets four hourly, and nausea for which he was using very little maxolon. I commenced him on a slow-release oral form of morphine (MS Contin) ostensibly for better control of his pain.

I had now seen Keith four times, and he was making a persistent request for assistance. However, I was having great difficulty in understanding him. He seemed quite fixated on ending his life now, and I could not persuade him to try to find some continuing purpose in his life—he seemed completely self-centred, oblivious of any needs his wife might have. To my surprise, and concern, she seemed to totally support his immediate need for death. He seemed unaware of the risks and difficulties involved in accomplishing what he wanted of me, or that what he wanted of me had apparently been 'refused' by three other treating doctors. Whilst I had assisted a number of people to deal with their end-of-life suffering in their own way, it had always been my aim to try to support them in a way that allowed them to go as far with their life as possible before bowing out.

Had it been legal and safe for me to prescribe barbiturates for him, I would at this point have sought a second medical opinion, but also a psychiatric opinion. In repeatedly asserting that he wished to end his life, he appeared to me to be denying any possibility of satisfaction in his own future. If treatable depression was not present I would have considered prescribing barbiturates. There is no doubt that a sufficient dose of oral, quick-acting barbiturates is the optimal way for a person with intolerable and unrelievable suffering to end their life. It is light years ahead of any other method. It will usually quickly cause deep sleep without fuss, and result in death within one half to two hours in most cases (depending on the type of barbiturate).

My aim was to continue to support him and gradually provide him with a sufficient supply of antidepressants, morphine and anti-emetic that would allow him to securely end his life if he determined that he could not continue. Determining what such a dose should be, however, is something of a guess. When I saw him again after another week, I prescribed more MS Contin, although his symptoms had not changed greatly, apart from further loss of weight. He needed to increase his maxolon (anti-emetic) to control his nausea.

Keith then failed to keep his planned weekly appointment. This disturbed me as I felt he was perhaps losing trust in me to deliver. He may not have been aware of how difficult it was for me to pre-scribe barbiturates at that time, and that I was struggling to find another way. I also felt that his suffering was not yet intolerable. I felt that Keith's physical symptoms were reasonably palliated, but had I underestimated the impact of his loss of appetite, weight and energy? Neil MacDonald and his palliative care colleagues from Canada had written about this:

Weight loss, asthenia and anorexia [loss of appetite], often associated with chronic nausea, are among the most common symptoms afflicting patients with advanced cancer … Family studies demonstrate that the cachexia-anorexia-asthenia complex ranks at the top of physical causes of suffering and contributes to psycho-social distress. The syndrome devastates family relations and makes the patient dependent on the family and health care institutions. As patients with cachexia-anorexia are often weak and unable to care for themselves, family resources are severely taxed, and patients often require institutional care for prolonged periods prior to death.[3]

Those comments usually apply to that stage when a patient is virtually confined to bed—Keith was not in this state yet (he probably still had about three months to live), but with his disease it would certainly come, and he knew it. Did I underestimate his psychological and existential suffering? At this stage of my experience I was not so aware of the powerful effect of such suffering. His only comment to me in this area was that he did not want to hang around for weeks or months during a long, drawn-out terminal illness, as he was unable to do those things that had given him pleasure in the past. We can all lose perspective when under stress—this is why second opinions are so valuable and necessary.

When I phoned Keith's wife to enquire about him, I was not entirely surprised to find out that he had already taken his life. She was critical of my lack of help! I was concerned that obviously both she and her husband had felt let down, and I wanted to learn more about his decision and about how I had failed to satisfy. I did not feel that this could be pursued usefully over the phone and arranged to meet her in a quiet place to discuss things. She agreed, but later phoned, leaving a message to cancel the meeting. I do not know whether he used the medication I prescribed to end his life. I certainly had not given him any specific instruction as to how to use it.

This was the first and only time that a person to whom I felt I had given a commitment to help had 'bailed out' before I had completed the 'agreement'. Looking back, I think he must have felt I was not committed or was ambivalent, as I had given him no specific advice. I have always been a strong supporter of the patient's autonomy in decision-making, particularly at the end of life, and believe that this should be respected. By the same token, the doctor involved in end-of-life decisions also has his autonomy to consider. He has a conscience that must be respected by the patient, and an ethical framework for his decisions. All legislation that has ever been seriously proposed for the legalisation of physician–assisted dying protects the doctor's right to refuse assistance on any ground (though he has a responsibility to inform his patient that there may be others who might assist in those circumstances). Thus the patient's autonomy is constrained by the need to find a doctor whose autonomy is in synchrony with their own, and it is almost certain the doctor will need to be convinced of a hopeless illness and significant suffering, which is otherwise unrelievable, before he will assist.

Suicide is usually an autonomous act that does not involve another person, but if a doctor is to be involved, his autonomy must also be considered. There may need to be some compromise of autonomy on the part of the patient in physician–assisted dying by self-administration. The same is true of the palliative care provision of terminal sedation, but this compromise can only be reached through open and honest dialogue between patient and doctor, and not by a unilateral decision by the doctor. The doctor should not use his power in the relationship to impose his choice of terminal sedation or refusal of food and fluids on his patient, as it is alleged has happened in the Netherlands. Dr Charles F McKhann, an American cancer surgeon, expresses this succinctly in his book *A Time to Die*:

> Autonomy also has limits that should be understood. Suicide,
> which is legal, is a private act. Because it requires no interaction

with anyone else, it is the only completely autonomous step that one can take to end one's life. A soon as a physician is included to assist in any way autonomy must be shared. The patient shares autonomy in finding a physician who is willing to help and in agreeing on terms, the timing and the method to be used. Regardless of whether assisted dying is legal or not, some negotiation with the physician will be necessary, and some compromise should be expected. She is not obliged to accept responsibility, and she is free to set her own requirements, including some form of public oversight. The confidential nature of the physician-patient relationship will necessarily be qualified. The invasion of privacy of both patient and physician is the unavoidable cost of legal approval and protection.[4]

I do not endorse euthanasia on demand. Requests have been made to me by distraught people when first learning they have cancer, but they need support to get through such a crisis, and I do not believe any doctor would accede to such a request without extensive work to overcome the probable depression associated with that request.

Keith's story highlights the unsatisfactory nature of covert euthanasia practice which makes the referral for second opinion such a difficult matter. For a second opinion from a palliative care specialist or psychiatrist to be of value, the individual's choice for euthanasia must be revealed, but this immediately creates possible legal difficulties for both doctors.

It was clear to me that there were communication problems in our relationship. Either Keith was not communicating the depth of his suffering to me, or I was not hearing him. Alternatively, I was not giving him sufficient confidence and support for him to continue with his life. There was no doubt that my relationship with Keith was affected by a sense of fear and anxiety on my part, and this is not conducive to the best communication. Whatever the reason, this was a failure that I deeply regret. I had a tendency to blame Keith for not understanding the problem, but in truth it was my responsibility as a doctor to guide the communication. It would have been avoidable in my view if the law had allowed a more open relationship, the involvement of other doctors, and a more certain outcome.

There is no doubt that medical practice involves relationships between people, and comfortable relationships are important in medicine as they are in all other walks of life. Without this, it is difficult to fully understand the nature of the problem. Nowhere is this more important than when trying to convey the presence and extent of existential suffering. Not all doctors are sensitive to existential suffering, or, if they are, do not believe it falls within their ambit for consideration or treatment. This is strange as existential suffering is intimately involved in all psychological medicine. When existential suffering is related to disease of great severity, it forms part of what is often called a 'total pain syndrome', in which the physical, psychological, emotional and existential are inextricably involved. Whilst the physical suffering may be obvious, the existential may be hidden, particularly if the person is not able to, or not encouraged to, express it fully. It requires empathy, to put oneself in the patient's position, to understand just what is behind the not so obvious suffering, and it requires subtle dialogue to encourage clear expression of concerns. Even then, as with Keith, it is possible to underestimate the position. The involvement of other doctors in the dialogue might have altered our confused relationship.

12

A REPORTABLE DEATH?

*'The period leading to death is characterized by increasing prevalence
and severity of a multitude of physical, psychological, existential
and social problems.'*[1]
Dr Nathan Cherny, Palliative Care physician, Israel

*'The purpose of terminal sedation is to ease the suffering of the patient
and comply with his wishes; and the actual cause of death is the
administration of heavy doses of lethal substances. The same intent and
causation may exist when a doctor complies with a patient's request for
lethal medication to hasten death.'*
Justice Sandra Day O'Connor, US Supreme Court

In 1995 I had two reasons for seeking the opinion of the coroner
about the need to report deaths associated with terminal sedation.
These two reasons were interrelated. The first reason followed from my
view that a strict interpretation of the *Coroners Act 1985* (Vic) would
require many deaths associated with terminal sedation to be reported
to the coroner. I felt it was highly likely this was not occurring. The

person legally responsible for reporting the death was the doctor who had ordered the drugs which had hastened the death. That represented a significant conflict of interest. Further, there are penalties for failing to report a reportable death. The doctor who fails to report a reportable death may not only suffer a financial penalty but may also be suspected of 'burying the evidence'. Uncertainty in the operation of the law in this important area is not acceptable.

More important than this aspect, however, is the question of giving doctors the confidence to use terminal sedation for terminally ill patients and to make all doctors aware that this practice is acceptable. Doctors should not be in fear of providing maximum relief of pain and suffering as stated by the *Medical Treatment Act 1988* (Vic), even if it hastens death. I was sure that this practice was as secret to many practitioners as it had been to me prior to 1997 when I discovered it by accident. I felt that it was important that this matter was discussed in an open manner, not secretively as alluded to by Ventafridda[2] and as appeared to be commonplace, and that a clear statement by the coroner would help.

My second reason for wanting guidance from the legal authorities was that I could see the very real possibility that I might personally face the question of providing terminal sedation. Statements that I had made to the media, particularly in 1995, about helping patients to die, resulted in requests from more than my fair share of patients who wanted a hastened death. Providing maximum relief from pain and suffering may result in the hastening of death when using terminal sedation. If this situation arose, I wanted to know my precise rights and responsibilities under the law. My correspondence with the coroner and Attorney-General left me in no doubt that the matter was unclear and that they were not prepared to clarify it, but it was my view that under a strict interpretation of the *Coroners Act*, a report of such a death was the correct action.

My concern was realised in July 1997, following a phone call from a 63-year-old widow, Pamela, who had been ill for only five weeks.

Lower abdominal and back pain had led to a colonoscopy that revealed an obstructing bowel cancer. An operation confirmed that the cancer was widespread throughout the abdominal cavity and liver, and the disease was incurable. The primary cancer could not be removed, so a bowel bypass was performed to relieve her obstruction. Five injections of chemotherapy did nothing to slow the progress of this cancer and, as is so often the case, produced its own significant morbidity. Her abdomen filled rapidly with ascites (fluid produced in the abdominal cavity due to the irritation of the cancer) causing her abdomen to resemble a late pregnancy. Two and a half and then 4 litres of fluid were removed via a needle but the fluid relentlessly reformed with no relief. Her appetite vanished and her weight plummeted, with a corresponding loss of energy. The physical devastation and psychological disintegration caused by this virulent cancer was astonishing. She was taking a large amount of morphine orally per day with reasonable control of her pain, but her pain was not the predominant issue. Her quality of life was spiralling out of control, her personhood was being stripped away, and it could only get rapidly worse.

I listened quietly to Pamela's story, asking a few questions to expand the picture and understand the depth of her suffering, and to search for indications of depression. She was already being treated for depression, but although she had a severely depressed mood, it was not out of proportion to her disastrous situation. She had the support of an attentive general practitioner, an excellent cancer and palliative care specialist, and was receiving home palliative care help, yet she was asking me for help to end her life. I empathised with her and said I respected her right to have her suffering properly relieved. I explained her rights under the *Medical Treatment Act*, indicating she had the right to refuse further chemotherapy and aspiration of abdominal fluid, and that she could ask for more aggressive relief of her symptoms. She had not discussed the depth of her distress with her treating doctors, a common communication failure in these situations, so I advised her to do so, but left open the option of ringing me again if she was not satisfied with her care. I was reluctant to get involved, and hoped that her treating doctors would, after appropriate discussion, agree to provide maximum relief of pain and suffering. That was their responsibility, but they did not. Perhaps her request frightened them, as it did me.

I was not surprised when she rang me again a week later, having deteriorated further. Her palliative care was not providing adequate relief, and she was desperate. Since I had only talked to her by phone, it was essential that I should meet her to better understand her. Her daughter brought her to my office in a wheelchair, and her suffering was almost palpable as she entered the room. Her face was haggard and pale, the loss of weight clearly etched. Her abdomen protruded massively as if she was pregnant. I reconfirmed the details of her story. Despite taking a large dose (200 mg) of morphine daily she still had constant abdominal discomfort with sharper intermittent pains. She had constant nausea and no appetite, and had considerable weight loss despite the accumulation of fluid in her abdomen. This caused extreme weakness and she had difficulty walking. She was breathless on the slightest exertion. Her bowels were still working with the aid of a laxative. She was drowsy for much of the time, probably because of the morphine, her antidepressant and her sedative. She was also taking cortisone.

I needed to examine her to confirm the diagnosis, but I felt guilty as I observed her distress as she struggled to climb onto the examination couch. The extreme exhaustion of someone with such a cancer can be easily underestimated if one merely observes them in repose. Her abdomen was tense and grossly distended, as though she was nine months pregnant, but instead of a smooth well-covered abdomen, I found wasted tightly stretched skin with visible nodularity, which corresponded with large tumour masses palpable in her abdomen. Fluid collection completed the distension. On examining her chest, I detected evidence of probable collections of fluid in the chest cavities on both sides that were contributing to her breathlessness.

Pamela was obviously severely distressed. She had many symptoms of depression (which were also common symptoms of her disease), but she was already receiving treatment for it. To my mind, her emotional state was proportional to her situation. At the most she had two weeks to live and no further psychiatric therapy could possibly alter her mind in that time and in the face of a crescendo of physical symptoms.

The rapid progress of Pamela's cancer was astonishing. What I have not described, and which cannot be measured, was her psychological and existential distress. Two months ago she was well, enjoying life and looking to the future. Now her only 'future' was of gross and increasing suffering. Every day was worse than the previous one; her personality was being consumed by her disease and drugs, and she could see no dignity in the progressive disintegration of her sense of self. She was being ably supported by her family and her health carers, but she had symptoms that are impossible to palliate by any means. She had some pain, but it was the least of her problems—whilst it could be further diminished, this would be achieved only at the expense of further drowsiness and confusion. Three other symptoms—her weakness, her breathlessness and her existential distress—were not capable of palliation in any way except by her being rendered unconscious, as by terminal sedation.

She had sent me the following letter:

I have decided to end my life because of the hopelessness and unbearable disease I have. I have had a wonderful life up until now and do not wish to continue my life any further as the end is inevitable.

This decision has been discussed with others in a general way but the final decision is entirely mine—I have given it a great deal of thought. I have recently become a member of the Euthanasia Society of Victoria and I agree with its credo. I have made the decision alone—no one has helped me. I have made a 'will' and 'Power of Attorney for Health Care'.

If I am discovered before I have stopped breathing, I forbid
anyone, including doctors or paramedics, to attempt to revive me.
If I am revived, I shall sue anyone who aided in this.

She was asking me for physician-assisted dying by providing her with
medication or injection. Because she was vomiting intermittently and
probably had a low-grade bowel obstruction, ending her life by oral
means was unpredictable. I told her that it was illegal to deliberately
help her to end her life, but that I believed it was not illegal to palliate
her symptoms in an aggressive manner, even if such treatment hastened
her death. I explained that she could refuse all further treatment and I
could give her continuous morphine and sedatives to completely relieve
her suffering so that she would sleep until she died. Clearly the provision of fluids would significantly prolong her dying and I advised that
I would not provide them by artificial means, with which she agreed.
I also warned her and her daughter that I would almost certainly have
to report her death to the coroner and of the consequences of that for
them. Because this was a very significant decision for her and one that
should be given careful consideration, I suggested that she and her
daughter discuss the matter overnight and call me in the morning if
they wanted my further care.

Her daughter rang me early the next morning to say that she had
deteriorated overnight with further pain and some vomiting, and
requested that I treat her mother. I arranged her admission to hospital
and rang her GP who confirmed the clinical details and indicated that
he had been told by her oncologist there was nothing further he could
do for her except provide terminal care. In hospital she completed a
Refusal of Treatment Certificate and requested 'complete relief of pain
and distress with appropriate analgesia and sedation'. Pamela was clearly
suffering from a crescendo of suffering that is often referred to in
palliative care literature as death approaches, and so I immediately
commenced treatment with morphine and a sedative (midazolam) via
a continuous infusion under the skin. The aim was to completely relieve

her pain and to cause her to sleep continuously to palliate her physical and existential suffering. The assessment of the minimum necessary dosage to achieve this for any given individual is an arbitrary matter and is often achieved only by observation. Commonly in conventional palliative care, an arbitrarily selected low dose is given from which base incremental increases are made until optimal palliation is achieved. As with the prostate cancer sufferer (chapter 9), this may take some days, during which time the patient certainly does not have maximum relief of pain and suffering. It is my belief that, if sedation is necessary for a dying person, it should be set immediately at a level that provides maximum relief.

The dose I chose made her sleep for nearly twenty-four hours, but when she woke it was discovered that her infusion needle had become displaced. Unfortunately she had severe pain and vomited faecal fluid (dark foul-smelling intestinal fluid, often indicative of bowel obstruction). Pamela and her daughter were gravely distressed by this unexpected event, as I was. I was now very concerned that her bowel obstruction was increasing and that there was a risk of her vomiting while she was unconscious and dying through the inhalation of vomit, a truly tragic, undignified and unacceptable end. It was now imperative that this dying process not be prolonged. Immediate further injections of morphine and sedative were given, together with a significant increase in the ongoing dosage for the continuous infusion. She then slept for a further twenty-four hours before she woke again in great distress and delirium and attempted to get out of bed. This greatly upset her daughter, who was sleeping in the bed beside her. Immediate drug treatment rendered her unconscious until she died three hours later.

This was the first time I had used terminal sedation as a primary palliative treatment, associated with the non-provision of food and fluids, and the outcome was not satisfactory to me, Pamela or her daughter. First, none of us anticipated or wished for her to wake in delirium on two occasions. In retrospect, I had relied too heavily on morphine and given too little sedation. I had not realised how deep the sedation had to be, and was not then aware of the advice of Professor Robert Twycross, in the *Oxford Textbook of Palliative Medicine*, that inadequate sedation may make things worse.[3] It was a mistake I vowed never to make again. Second, in my haste to relieve her suffering, I had initiated sedation before her daughter had had the opportunity to say a final 'goodbye'. I had presumed that this important event had already occurred, but in fact it had not, to her daughter's regret. Another step on the learning curve.

Once again, I had assisted in hastening the death of my patient on request. This occurred through the provision of deep sedation with the intention to palliate her suffering. The withholding of fluids, which were not clinically indicated, added a significant contribution due to dehydration. The intention to palliate became associated with the intention to hasten death in order to prevent the disaster of death by inhalation of vomit. Pamela suffered a crescendo of pain and suffering as she neared the end of her life. In response this requires a parallel increase in palliative treatment to stay in front of this enormous challenge. It fully justifies the use of deep sedation maintained until death occurs, and this is what I attempted to do.

Palliative care expert Dr David J Roy made this observation in an editorial for the *Journal of Palliative Care*: 'Those who argue for the ethical and legal justification of euthanasia must wonder about the clarity or the arbitrariness of the distinction between inducing unconsciousness and rapidly terminating life, if and when dying persons experience a crescendo of unmanageable suffering in the last days of life'.[4]

You might not be surprised that I agree.

I duly rang the coroner's office to report her death, only to hear the coroner's assistant say, 'Doc, these cases are not usually reported'. I replied that it was precisely for that reason I was reporting the matter! My deposition to the coroner stated that the reason for reporting the death was 'death associated with drug excess', and that a contributory cause of death was 'drug-induced coma'. Unbeknown to me, her daughter had objected to an autopsy. This objection was respected and on the basis of inspection of the body, the forensic pathologist stated, 'there is no evidence to suggest that death was due to other than natural causes', and found that the most likely cause of death was 'disseminated carcinoma of the colon'. It was as though the last two days of her life had not occurred.

I discovered this pathologist's report accidentally when I was photocopying Pamela's medical record some six weeks later. A copy of the report was in her hospital file, yet I, the reporting doctor, had received no such advice. I wrote to the coroner's office requesting a copy of this report, only to receive a reply stating that 'this report is not yet available'. This was typical of the obfuscation that occurred over the next twelve months as I attempted to find out whether this death was reportable, both from the coroner and the Attorney-General. Despite having reported the death on the grounds of possible 'death associated with drug excess', I had not been interviewed by the Coroner's Office. Despite being the reporting doctor, I had not received any information from the coroner on the matter despite five letters of request and, similarly, had received no response as to whether the death was or was not reportable.

Section 18 of the *Coroners Act 1985* (Vic) states:

(1) If a person asks a coroner to hold an inquest into a death which
   a coroner has jurisdiction to investigate, the coroner may—
(a) hold an inquest or ask another coroner to do so; or
(b) refuse the request and give reasons in writing for the refusal
   to the person and to the State Coroner within seven days after
   receiving the request.

This seemed to be the only way in which I could force the coroner to address the matter, so on 10 September 1998 (after contacting Pamela's daughter, explaining my reasons and obtaining her consent) I formally requested the State Coroner hold an inquest into the death. No refusal was forthcoming within seven days, so presumably an inquest was under way! On 4 December 1998 I was interviewed by the coroner's assistant. Nearly three years later, on 12 September 2001, I received a final letter from the coroner that stated, 'Her death has been found to have been from natural causes and therefore is not a reportable death pursuant to the *Coroners Act*'. Thus it had taken more than four years for the coroner to reluctantly deliver this decision. Pity the poor doctor on the spot who has to make an instant decision about this question regarding his just-deceased patient.

A death 'from natural causes' in 1997 therefore was one in which a person expressed the intention to end their life because of their 'hopelessness and unbearable disease', and requested assistance to do so. That person could be fully informed and rational, be receiving medical treatment that deliberately put them into a coma with the intention of maintaining that coma without any other medical support until they died, thus hastening their death.

In the course of his four-year investigation into Pamela's death, the coroner had sought an expert opinion regarding my actions. Whether by design or accident, that opinion was obtained from a palliative care specialist who happened to be a vigorous opponent of voluntary euthanasia (not necessarily the case for all such doctors). Her report was critical in minute detail of the drugs and the dosage of drugs that I had used, and implied that a different course would have followed in her care, but she could not find that the terminal sedation was ill-advised. In her view, my 'attempts to induce sedation and possibly respiratory depression by increased analgesia did not conclusively result in an early death'. The coroner kindly passed her report on to the Medical Practitioners Board of Victoria who initiated an inquiry into my practice. Their conclusion was: 'The Board considered that your treatment choices were not unreasonable in the circumstances and found that there was no evidence that you had been unprofessional in your conduct towards [Pamela]'.

I was gratified and relieved by this Medical Board decision. I had fully anticipated the coroner's decision, but was mystified as to why it had taken so long. Clearly, terminal sedation was a legal option for relieving suffering while hastening death, but before this decision was made known I was faced with two further dilemmas (see chapters 13 and 14).

I referred to the learning curve when I neglected to ensure that Pamela could say goodbye to her daughter. Due to the covert nature of physician-assisted dying in Victoria, I had to learn how to provide best practice on the job. There were no colleagues with whom I could consult. There were no detailed references to consult, books by experienced doctors to read, or training courses to attend. I had to learn the importance of thoroughly researching the palliative care literature to learn about terminal sedation, as it was not reported in the routine medical literature. As the palliative care physician Ventafridda said, 'it was rarely discussed in an open fashion'. I had to discover the best medication to use, and its effects. I needed contacts in the Netherlands for this information. Furthermore, I had to learn about counselling, and what was and was not possible through palliative care. I doubt that most doctors would have had the time or inclination to do this research. I have no doubt that when physician-assisted dying is legalised, it will be essential to establish extensive educational and training programs for doctors who want to provide such treatment. In the Netherlands, they have established a mentor scheme (SCEN—Support and Consultation in the Netherlands). This involves a panel of doctors who have been trained and have experience in the proper implementation of physician-assisted dying, who act as an expert referral source for either formal second opinion or informal advice. These specially trained doctors meet regularly to discuss issues and problems that arise. Such an organised approach is essential in any country where physician-assisted dying might be legalised to ensure that good practice is the result. I would be the first to admit that bad practice is possible if doctors are not properly trained or ignore proper guidelines, but this is even more likely where no training, guidelines or law exist.

13

IS THIS THE BEST WE CAN DO?

'The principle of autonomy is the dominant ethic of health care in North America and Western Europe.'[1]

Dr Douglas Martin, L Emanuel, PA Singer

15 September 1998

I write to seek your help, having very carefully considered and pondered over my situation. I am a resident in the above nursing home, here for two years so far, being a victim of multiple sclerosis.

I have now reached a stage where I can no longer help myself, being 'locked' into a wheelchair, and the paralysis now reaching both hands, after total paralysis of my legs.

As you can well imagine, my future is very bleak, with little or no quality of life. Whilst I am receiving loving care on the part of all the staff here, I just feel there's nothing left in life to continue. Thus, I write appealing to you to advise and help to end a situation over which I no longer have any control.

Please help me.

Yours sincerely,

X

Note.

The above has been dictated to me by 'Jane' bearing her mark.

Doris ....

By now, I had sufficient experience of people with chronic progressive or permanent neurological disease to understand the implications of this situation. I had spent almost thirty years treating patients with extensive paralysis due to spinal injuries at the Austin Hospital in Melbourne as a urological consultant to the Spinal Injury Unit. I was well aware of the extraordinary challenge that paraplegia, and more significantly quadriplegia, presented and the enormous courage that these, usually young, people brought to bear on their problem. But the more extensive the paralysis, the greater the problem. For quadriplegics (who cannot move any limb), who may also depend upon a ventilator to breathe for them, the suffering can be intolerable. One such unfortunate patient, John McEwen, by his refusal of continuing ventilator support, created a controversy and debate that ultimately helped in the passage of the Victorian *Medical Treatment Act*. As I mentioned earlier, this Act created a statutory confirmation of the existing common law right that allowed any competent adult to refuse treatment, even though such refusal of treatment would hasten, or actually cause, their death.

Jane had a different problem. Her condition would certainly get slowly worse, but she was unlikely at any time to have any treatment that she could refuse. Multiple sclerosis does not cause respiratory failure. To paraphrase her words, 'I am a victim, locked into a wheelchair, in a situation over which I no longer have any control'.

It had become abundantly clear to me that the problems faced by people with a chronic, progressive, unrelenting neurological disease were far greater than those faced by a person with terminal cancer. These people have a hopeless illness (incurable but with no discernable end-point) rather than a terminal illness. Yet virtually all the public arguments about physician-assisted dying are focused on relieving the suffering due to pain from terminal cancer.

It is true that much of the pain of terminal cancer can be relieved or minimised by good palliative care, and it is uncommon for someone in this state not to be treated with narcotics at the end of life. It is equally true, according to Dr M Levy, writing on the 'Pharmacological treatment of cancer pain' in the prestigious *New England Journal of Medicine*, that 'cancer pain can be effectively treated in 85–95% of patients' and that 'in the final days of life, pain not controlled by therapies aimed at both comfort and function can be relieved by intentional sedation'.[2] And yet, pain is not the most common reason that some people request physician-assisted dying. Other physical symptoms, such as breathlessness, cachexia (loss of appetite, weight and energy), loss of control of bodily functions (incontinence) and the accompanying indignity, are also significant. So are emotional, psychological and existential suffering. The noted Australian Palliative Care Professor Michael Ashby summed this up when he said, 'For many people who are dying it is not just a question of comfort or absence of physical suffering but a loss of function, independence and role which are hardest to bear'.[3] On another occasion, he wrote: 'However, the idea that modern palliative care can relieve all the suffering associated with death and dying is a flawed approach'.[4] Roger Hunt, another palliative care specialist, put it this way: 'The hospice ideal of providing a pain-free comfortable and dignified death is usually unachievable and should not be promised.'[5] Jane summed up her losses of function and independence as a 'loss of control'. Of all the reasons for requests for medical assistance in dying, the desire for control is the most common and the most profound.

My first visit to Jane was in September 1998, and thus began an intense 8-month relationship that ended with her death. She was fifty-two, and had first been diagnosed with multiple sclerosis at the age of forty, although, in retrospect, she could recognise the first symptoms some years earlier. Her first symptoms involved tiredness and weakness in the legs and difficulty walking. Unlike the more common form of MS, her disease was progressive and without remissions and fluctuations. Her bladder function deteriorated so that she became incontinent and had to have a permanent urethral catheter (a tube into her bladder). Four years earlier, she had become affected in the left arm, which was now totally paralysed, and then her right arm and hand started becoming weak.

For the past five years, she had been confined to a wheelchair, and had been cared for by her loving sister and her family, until this became impossible in the home environment. She was fortunate that her sight was not affected (a common problem in MS). Her breathing and speech were normal.

She suffered moderate pain in her joints, which had become stiff because she could not use them. She had pain in her pressure areas due to her inability to move even one centimetre to relieve such pressure from prolonged immobility. With good care, however she had only minor pressure ulcers. She suffered painful muscle spasms in her legs and body, which had fortunately been greatly relieved by a baclofen (anti-spasmodic) pump. She used only occasional sedatives and analgesics, preferring to put up with the chronic pain rather than become reliant on medication. She could sit in her wheelchair only if she was restrained in it, and could not change her position at any time without help. She could not feed herself, she could not empty her bladder (hence the catheter) and could not use her bowels, requiring someone else to perform manual evacuations.

Despite all this, by extreme good fortune, she could still do one thing of critical importance to her. She could still paint.

Jane had been a significant artist in her earlier days, having won awards and having had exhibitions. Despite the weakening of her right arm and hand, she continued to paint with watercolours, attending a weekly class and showing her work. This continuing ability to create was her life's defining influence. Sadly, her ability to use her hand was fast declining. She showed me some of her recent work, which, despite her disability, had great charm and quality in its simplicity. I could understand how important this mode of expression was to her, and her anguish at seeing her facility fade. I could understand why she had reached the point of ultimate decision.

As her ability to paint disappeared, Jane's view of her life was that it had become almost devoid of pleasure. Was this anhedonia a manifestation of depression, or of reality? What was left? Her life was one of suffering in the broadest sense, characterised by total dependence and almost without meaning. She saw her life as close to its useful end, and she was ready to leave it but she lacked the means to do this. In desperation she sought my advice.

My immediate response was to try to convey my sympathetic understanding of her situation and her request, and to indicate that I would support her and hope to find a way to assist her in a very difficult situation. This could involve an extended dialogue to develop a mutual understanding, and would need to involve her family. She had discussed these matters with her devoted sister, who, however, did not support her intention to end her life. I encouraged her to continue with that dialogue. Jane was being treated by several doctors, including a general practitioner, a rehabilitation specialist and a surgeon who had performed a mastectomy for breast cancer earlier that year. They were giving her good care, but none of them was open to discussing ways of helping her in the way she had asked me.

I continued to see Jane regularly at weekly intervals over the next four months. She was highly intelligent, widely read and a joy to visit. I learnt a great deal about her and her beliefs and values, and I could understand even better why she wanted to end her life. She had been married, but had separated from her husband. She had no children, but she was very close to her sister. She had a Christian upbringing, but now held no firm religious beliefs, although she showed interest in Buddhist philosophy. Once having made her request for help, it was not constantly repeated in a demanding manner, but it was clear from our frequent conversations that her intention never wavered.

I found her to be utterly rational. Despite her distressing circumstances, she seemed to be in a state of grace and mental repose, so long as she could paint. I saw my role as supporting her for as long as possible. We talked about many things, and I brought her *Tuesdays with Morrie*,[6] which we read together. This is an inspirational book relating the dialogue between a journalist and his old philosophy professor, who is dying of MND. It reveals how, even in significant adversity, people may find fulfilling avenues of creativity whilst waiting for the moment to depart.

I am a keen bird-watcher and brought Jane photos of some of my favourite birds for her to paint for me. Her simple yet exquisite results are among my treasured possessions. This was but one of the many ways I explored to help her to find meaning in her life. She was involved in a documentary for Danish television, and an interview and article in *The Age*.[7] Unfortunately, there was only one other inmate of the nursing home with whom she could have a conversation, but that only seemed to occur if she listened and he talked!

Jane presented me with a dilemma. She was making a rational and persistent request for my assistance to end her life. She explained that her existence had become one of intolerable suffering due to her hopeless illness, which was largely existential, although it also had some physical elements. Unlike Pamela, she had no severe pain that would allow me to readily deliver narcotics and sedation whilst withholding food and fluids. I found her request compelling, so I committed to helping her. Finding a solution, however, was extremely difficult. Providing assistance in suicide for able-bodied people is relatively simple, involving the provision of medication together with the advice on how to use it, after an appropriate dialogue and support through the decision-making period. Jane, however, was completely unable to prepare and ingest medication without help, and somebody would have to do this for her. Moreover, her nursing home was a public environment where it was impossible to guarantee the privacy needed to help her; nor was it possible to guarantee protection from interference which might foil her intention. In short, it was impossible, because of her physical condition and her living circumstances, to assist her safely and without clear legal danger to those who would be intimately associated with that assistance. Even if she were to leave the nursing home on a temporary basis, the circumstances of her death would create a dangerous position for those who were caring for her at the time.

In early 1999, I became aware of an article published by Dr Linda Emanuel in the *Journal of the American Medical Association* entitled 'Facing requests for physician–assisted suicide'. As a doctor who opposes voluntary euthanasia by lethal injection or patient self-administration, Emanuel described an approach that would deflect such requests, offering the alternative of patient refusal of oral intake of food and fluids in specific circumstances. She argued that her approach was based on two generally uncontested arguments:'that individuals can reject unwanted interventions, and that suffering individuals have a legitimate claim to comfort care'.[8] Essentially, she was arguing that, in certain circumstances, it was better and more moral to encourage someone to cease taking oral hydration, rather than for the physician to accede to the patient's request for assisted suicide. She stated that such management would 'offer thereby a similar degree of relief from physical suffering as induced death but without the higher degree of moral questioning associated with physician–assisted suicide'. She acknowledged that 'while patients may continue for days in this state before dying, the patient is not suffering'. Whilst I strongly disagreed with Emanuel's central philosophy (the immorality of assisted suicide), I realised that her proposition would be applicable to Jane's situation. The Victorian *Medical Treatment Act* allowed people to refuse medical treatment but not palliative care, which was defined as (a) the provision of reasonable medical procedures for the relief of pain, suffering and discomfort; or (b) the reasonable provision of food and water. I regarded the provision of food and water by artificial means (intravenous or tube) as medical treatment that could be refused by a competent person such as Jane, and it is most certainly accepted as against all civilised customs to force-feed any rational person by oral means. It seems clear that in these circumstances, a patient could expect a doctor to relieve any suffering caused by their refusal of food and fluids. This proposition hinged on the request being rational and the person being competent to make such a request.

The concept of voluntary withdrawal of food and fluids as a means of ending suffering has been discussed with increasing frequency over the past ten years. Most writers accept the patient's right to refuse any treatment, even if that will result in their death. Gert and colleagues spelt this out very clearly:

> Overruling a competent patient's refusal of treatment, including life-preserving treatment always involves depriving the patient of freedom, and usually causes pain. No impartial person would publicly allow these kinds of paternalistic actions and so they are morally unacceptable ... When patients have terminal diseases, however, it is generally the case when they want to die, it is rational for them to choose death.[9]

Although most medical authors were not prepared to discuss terminal dehydration and its palliation, a few brave souls did. Cherny and colleagues pointed out in 1996 that 'In patients who are cognitively intact, dehydration can precipitate delirium and diminish interactional function'.[10]

JL Bernat, a pre-eminent American neurologist, was forthright in his view. He wrote that:

> Physicians caring for patients dying of refusal of hydration and nutrition have an important responsibility to provide adequate symptom control ... Physicians should be willing to prescribe narcotics and benzodiazepines (sedatives) in dosages sufficient to abate

pain and other unpleasant sensations. They should not incorrectly limit the dosage of their prescriptions for fear of accelerating death; the intent should be to maintain adequate comfort during dying ... There needs to be societal acceptance that physicians have a moral duty to respect the rational wishes of competent chronically ill but not terminally ill patients who wish to die by valid refusals of therapy. There is no reason why such patients should not have the same rights as the terminally ill to refuse life sustaining therapies including hydration and nutrition.[11]

I was not aware of this view when I advised Jane, but I fully concurred when my research subsequently discovered it.

When I explained to Jane that she could end her life by ceasing to drink, she was horrified, until I explained that I would provide her with sedation upon her request. Such sedation would make her sleep during any distress that was caused by her action. After we discussed this in detail on a number of occasions, she accepted the idea. Meanwhile, her sister had approached me, indicating that she had come to accept the reality of Jane's situation, realising that her continued opposition was unfair to Jane and would only prolong her suffering. Although I did not have the faintest doubt about Jane's competence and rationality, I felt it would be wise to seek a psychiatric opinion, which was as follows:

Jane is surprisingly little disturbed in her mental state. She seems to be cognitively intact, with good memory, has insight, and no evidence of psychosis.

As far as depression is concerned, she has little or no evidence of a significant mood disorder. She does not appear sad, or even dispirited, she does not report any significant depressed mood, has only very occasional feelings of tension, sleeps reasonably well, enjoys her food, has a normal interest in her surroundings and in other people, and although she once criticised herself for staying with a man and perhaps adversely affecting her health, currently that is behind her and she has no pessimism, except in regard to continue to slowly deteriorate in her physical functioning.

She has difficulty in concentrating on reading, but that is because her eyes tend to wander. The only symptom related to depression from which she suffers is a wish 'for it all to be over', and in the circumstances of her progressive disablement, with no hope of recovery, I would regard that as an appropriate emotion.

Over the next few weeks, as her right arm and hand became weaker, it became clear that Jane was now ready, as she put it, 'to meet her maker'. We arranged a meeting at her sister's home, with Jane, her sister and her sister's husband and me. I explained, in clear detail, why and how the proposed course of action would unfold. Surprisingly, it was not a morbid occasion, but one at which Jane's natural humour and good spirits bubbled over, so happy was she to have some control over her future. I had explained that I would need to report her death to the coroner for two reasons. First, I had not had any reply from the coroner regarding my earlier use of terminal sedation and, second, that the circumstances under which I would be treating her were possibly unique in Victoria, and I did not want to be accused of hiding the truth. In my view, it was essential that the coroner comment on the process. All were agreed that I should do that.

On the agreed day, Jane entered hospital, having already stopped eating and drinking for two days. She had some complaint of loin pain, which I considered might be due to kidney infection. She completed a Refusal of Treatment Certificate, which indicated that she refused all treatment including provision of artificial fluid administration, and requested maximum relief of pain and suffering. I had already discussed and cleared my treatment care plan with the Director of Nursing. After two and a half days of refusing fluids, she requested me to provide sedation and pain relief. I commenced a continuous subcutaneous infusion of morphine (60 mg/24 hours) and midazolam (a short acting sedative, 40 mg/24 hours). She slept for the next eighteen hours, but then awoke; distressed at being awake, she requested more sedation. The midazolam dose was doubled, but six hours later she was again alert and distressed and requested more sedation. The midazolam dose was doubled again. Throughout the next twenty-four hours she was intermittently restless, and her sister, who was authorised as Jane's medical enduring power of attorney, requested more sedation. The midazolam was increased again, but it was not until the third day of sedation, when the dose of morphine was increased to 90 mg/24 hours and the midazolam to 360 mg/24 hours, that she remained continuously unconscious until she died some four days later.

Jane had endured two days without food and fluids before she asked for sedation. She slept fitfully and incompletely over the next three days whilst the sedative and narcotic dose was incrementally increased, and then remained in a deep, drug-induced coma for a further four days. She had managed to end her life, which she wanted, but was it as she wished? During the short periods of consciousness that occurred after the sedation commenced she clearly had some distress, but it was short-lived. I am sure that she did not fully envisage the consequences of a process that would take nine days (although I had advised her and her family that it could take from seven to fourteen days) and involve significant stress on her family and friends. They repeatedly asked me why it was taking so long and were clearly distressed. She did not die alone, as there were constant family and friends keeping a vigil at her bedside, communicating with her and comforting her. But as the days dragged by in what I can only describe as a thoroughly distasteful and, to me, undignified process, the stress that we all went through (family, friends, nurses and me) was heavy. I had not been involved in such a process before and had not fully comprehended that the time taken would involve so much anguish. I wished to speed up the process, but the rationale for treatment was the palliation of suffering due to the refusal of fluids, and hence I had to rely on medications for sedation rather than on medications for pain relief. I still felt justified in using small doses of morphine to relieve her pain due to her joints, pressure areas, kidney pain and hunger pains, but the principal reason for sedation was to relieve the psychological and emotional pain as well as the physical symptoms of dehydration. Now, upon reflection, I ought to have used a larger initial dose of midazolam. Yet, too large an initial dose might have increased my risk of being accused of intending to cause death rather than to palliate.

Fear of inappropriate accusation haunts all physicians who wish to provide adequate palliation with analgesics and sedatives, as it is only through the failure of a reasonable empirical dose to fully relieve the symptoms that a larger, again empirical, dose of medication can be used. Thus a 'stuttering', or gradual, approach to adequate palliation is far more common than an initial dose that will certainly relieve all suffering at the outset. When each failure of therapy occurs, the sedative dose can be increased. In Jane's case, each dose was doubled on proving inadequate, so that at the end, the dose of midazolam was nine times the initial dose.

Jane had achieved her aim, but in a way, and at a cost to others, that I believe she would not have wanted.

I remain highly ambivalent about this process—it did achieve its aim, but I question if it is an acceptable solution. As the process dragged on, I felt shame at my involvement in such a macabre process, and guilty that I had not had the courage to be more aggressive with the sedation, but in truth, I went as hard as I felt it was possible to do. In retrospect, I wish it had been possible to take a different road. Some patients do come to their own decision to cease food and fluids, and may not need large doses of medication for palliation, until close to the end. But Jane had only come to this decision on my advice, and with my assurance that she would not suffer at all. I felt a heavy burden of responsibility as to the outcome. Some may see it as dignified, but I did not.

Jane had requested my assistance in hastening her death, because she had a hopeless illness with chronic progressive paralysis that was nearing its end stage, and causing severe existential suffering. She elected to cause her death by refusing all food and fluids and I assisted her by providing sedation to palliate any additional suffering in this process. Unlike Pamela, where the drugs had hastened her death with minimal effect from the fluid absence, for Jane the principal cause of death, in my opinion, was dehydration, with the sedatives playing a secondary role.

I duly reported Jane's death to the coroner, and nervously waited for the Forensic Pathologist's report. This became available nearly four months after Jane's death. It contained the following statement:

> In providing the cause of death as given below I include those conditions or factors acting on [Jane] which in my opinion have caused her death or caused it to occur earlier than it might otherwise have done. This is a value-neutral exercise as far as I am concerned and it is not meant to imply endorsement or criticism of any aspect of [Jane's] management. Indeed, there is no reason for me to doubt that there was other than proper management of her condition pursuant to the completion of a 'Refusal of Treatment' certificate by [Jane's] Medical Power of Attorney. If there is any doubt about this, or any further evaluation of [Jane's] management is required, then the opinion of a palliative care specialist should be sought.
>
> In my opinion, the cause of death is:
> 1 Bronchopneumonia
> 1b Immobility in a woman with multiple sclerosis, refusing medical treatment and sustenance, managed with morphine and midazolam hastening the onset of unconsciousness (refusal of treatment certificate).

When I read this report, I was puzzled by three matters. Why was there no mention of dehydration? Jane had taken no fluids or food by mouth for nine days, and the only fluid that she did receive was the small amount of subcutaneous fluid used to dissolve and deliver the drugs. Her urine output chart indicated that for the last six days of her life, her output was considerably less per day than that which is necessary to maintain normal body chemistry and was typical of the normal response to lack of fluids. Second, there was no comment regarding the question of suicide, which I had raised in my report of the death to the coroner. Third, the toxicology report made no comment regarding the significance of the blood levels of morphine or midazolam. I therefore wrote to the pathologist seeking clarification of these matters.

After a prolonged correspondence with four letters back and forth, over eight months, the dog finally got his bone with this reply: 'I did not include dehydration in the conclusion as to the cause of death. I accept that this is a judgment call. If it was put to me that I should accept what was in the record about the volume of fluid consumed, then it would be reasonable to include dehydration in the cause of death'.

The coroner finally informed me in September 2001 of his opinions regarding the deaths of Pamela and Jane. Prior to this, however, in May 2000, I had reported another death through terminal sedation (Howard, chapter 14). Howard was suffering from cancer.

With respect to Jane, the coroner, in a 'finding without inquest', stated that the death was a reportable death 'because (the) pathologist determined that "factors acting on [Jane] which in my opinion have caused her death or caused it to occur earlier than it might otherwise have done"'.

This is an extraordinary statement—the deaths of Pamela and Howard both clearly occurred earlier than they might otherwise have done, yet they were not reportable. The difference between these situations, cancer on the one hand (Pamela and Howard) and chronic neurological disease (Jane) on the other, and the extent to which death occurred earlier than expected (days or weeks as opposed to months or years) is hardly sufficient to make a distinction between a reportable death and a natural death, when the proximate cause of the deaths is the same (namely sedation and dehydration), and in each case death occurred earlier than it might otherwise have done.

The coroner noted in his letter that the pathologist 'was not critical of your care' and also stated, 'As part of the investigation a report was sought from a palliative care expert, who was also not critical of your management'. He found that, 'It is not possible to say, on the evidence, whether the actions of Mr Syme hastened the eventual outcome'.

I received a copy of the report of the palliative care expert who advised the coroner (he was actually a neurologist). Some of his comments make interesting reading, as much for what he does not say or expand on, as what he does. He restricted his comments to the medical ethics of the case, and I was gratified by his comment: 'I cannot see any actions of Dr Syme which were unethical'.

His report stated:

> If I was the doctor looking after this woman when she made the request, I would have to check that she was not depressed in the sense of having a treatable psychosis and that she understood the implications of her decisions, but after being satisfied about these points I would feel a professional obligation to support her. I guess there would be doctors who had a religious commitment that made it impossible to support someone like [Jane] in this kind of situation but I think most doctors would offer support.

What intrigues me is why a religious commitment should alter the medical obligation to support, if the medical ethics are so clear. What judgement on religious grounds would deny support? Is it that a religious person is bothered by the possibility that death may have been hastened, or that assistance was rendered in suicide?

The report continued:

Once a doctor accepts that the patient's decision is a valid one
and that he has a professional obligation to support them, then,
the rest follows. One has to respect the orders about food, antibiotics etc. and one has to respect the request for 'aggressive relief
of pain and suffering'.

Medical ethics clearly allow a doctor to apply 'aggressive relief of pain
and suffering' at the request of the patient, yet it is surprising how some
doctors do not understand and apply this ethic.

The neurologist continued: 'Of course, the use of morphine and
midazolam may have slightly increased the speed with which [Jane] died
… Put another way, if the sedation had not been used, the death would
have been inevitable and might have been slightly slower but not that
much slower'.

There is recognition here that Jane's death was inevitable because
she took no food and fluids, although the use of the medication
may have hastened the death to a minor degree. Nevertheless, this
opinion clearly points to the significance of dehydration in the death,
a point the pathologist was at pains to try to avoid. There is a strange
dichotomy here between the opinion of the pathologist and the
clinician. The pathologist believed that death was principally due to
pneumonia associated with immobility (it would seem, due to the
unconsciousness caused by the drugs), and only very reluctantly
admitted that dehydration had an influence, whilst the clinician
believed that death would have occurred inevitably due to the lack
of fluids (which would not, of itself, have caused pneumonia), and that
whilst the drugs may have hastened death marginally, they were not
really significant. The coroner was happy to accept both opinions,
conflicting or not.

The neurologist's report continued:

It is uncommon for patients with multiple sclerosis to take this decision but it's not unknown. In most long term follow ups of multiple sclerosis suicide is a significant cause of death … In the circumstances where a person has no movement of any limb and no prospect of improvement, a decision to cease eating and drinking in order to die more quickly is understandable and not unreasonable.

The neurologist is clearly raising the question of suicide, as I did in my report of the death to the coroner. The neurologist clearly identified this as an act of suicide, and he clearly saw it as an utterly rational decision. The coroner, on the other hand, decided it was not suicide. Did he reach this conclusion because the act was rational, because of the method or, perhaps, for the sake of the family, as there is little benefit, but possibly harm, in calling such an action a suicide, bearing in mind the stigma such a descriptor carries? It was certainly not an act which the wider community would see as typical of suicide, yet there is no other word in the English language that fits these characteristics. Since this death occurred in relation to a Refusal of Treatment certificate, a valid document under the *Medical Treatment Act*, it is relevant to refer to the genesis of this Act.

The Parliamentary Committee of Inquiry that investigated dying with dignity in 1986, culminating in the *Medical Treatment Act* in 1988, considered the possible implication that refusal of treatment, which led to death, might be considered suicide. The Committee decided absolutely that it was not, and should not be seen in this way.[12] The Committee cited four principles that must be present for suicide to apply at common law. The first was that the person intending to commit suicide must actually die. The second principle was that the killer must deliberately intend to kill himself or herself and the third principle was that the person must have caused his or her own death. The fourth and final principle was that the first and second facts must happen at the same time. It was clear to me that these four principles were satisfied in Jane's case.

While the Committee's conclusion was probably reached to allow any person the freedom to refuse treatment without the stigma of suicide, and whilst many people might have no intention of using this refusal to deliberately hasten their deaths, it is undeniably true that some people with severe suffering and hopeless illness could take this decision with the explicit intent that they would cause their own death by such an action or inaction. If Jane had taken an overdose of drugs, it would have been described as suicide—but she could not. If she had shot herself, I presume it would have been described as suicide—but she could not. She could end her life only by ceasing to drink, but it was not considered to be suicide! She wanted her life to end, and was prepared to end her life, and took the only action that she could. The fact that this was a negative action, rather than positive, in no way alters the intent and the outcome. If someone deliberately jumps in front of a train it is suicide. Is it not also suicide if someone deliberately lies on the track and waits for the train to come by? Imagine a diabetic who is suffering the long-term complications of that disease. He has happily accepted treatment with insulin for some years, but is now losing his sight due to retinopathy, has lost control of his bladder due to neuropathy, has lost one leg and is threatened with the loss of the other because of vasculopathy. He decides that his quality of life is unacceptable and his suffering intolerable. If he deliberately injects an overdose of insulin to cause his death by hypoglycaemic (low blood sugar) coma, with the intention of ending his suffering, it would be considered suicide. If that same man deliberately refrains from injecting insulin and refuses further insulin, so that he dies of a hyperglycaemic coma (high blood sugar), is this not also suicide?

In 1992, the Catholic bioethicist Nicholas Tonti-Filipini described the death by withdrawal of treatment of a woman suffering from motor neurone disease.[13] A 45-year-old woman (Mrs N.) had fairly rapidly developed respiratory failure, leading to respiratory arrest and life support on a ventilator in a Catholic hospital. This occurred prior to the Parliamentary Committee of Inquiry that led to the *Medical Treatment Act*. It soon became clear that she had an atypical onset of MND when her limbs subsequently became paralysed. This woman was now ventilator dependent, paralysed, confined to bed and was not going to leave hospital. She made, according to Tonti-Filipini, frequent requests to the nursing staff 'to have the ventilator treatment withdrawn'. After discussions with the nursing staff, who had initially thought Mrs N. to be 'manipulative', her medical consultant (who strongly discouraged ceasing treatment), a barrister (the notorious Kevin Andrews, whose Federal Private Members' Bill scuppered Marshal Perron's world's first 1996 Northern Territory legislation allowing voluntary euthanasia), a psychiatrist (who found she was not mentally ill or being coerced), and Tonti-Filipini (who admirably supported the woman), all agreed that she had a moral right to refuse 'extremely burdensome treatment'.

What a strange turn of phrase, 'extremely burdensome treatment'— certainly not one that I had heard a patient utter spontaneously in more than twenty-five years consulting with patients who might have wished to refuse treatment. It smacks of the kind of jargon that Catholic theologians, barristers and bioethicists might find useful. A very convenient phrase if only it had been uttered by Mrs N. Much less challenging an answer to the question 'Why do you want the ventilator treatment withdrawn?' than 'because I want to die', or 'because I don't want to go on living in these circumstances'. These answers beg a further question, 'Why do you want to die?', to which the realistic response might be 'because I am now a burden to my family and I can no longer help to look after them'. It was also clear that Mrs N. greatly feared accidental disconnection or failure of the ventilator. However, we are not told, perhaps because she was not asked, that she felt she had no quality of life, that she had lost her independence, her role in life (as a wife and mother of two children) and possibly saw herself as a burden to her family. Whilst her family might predictably say that she was not a burden, the pragmatic reality was otherwise. Rational people know this—like Captain 'Titus' Oates, a member of Scott's Antarctic expedition, who, realising that he was holding up the group's progress, left the tent saying, 'I may be gone some time' and did not return. If Mrs N. was fully informed about switching off the ventilator, she would have known that she had two choices only—staying alive on the ventilator, or dying without it. Not very good choices admittedly, but she chose to die. She ultimately made a rational decision to die, not merely to be relieved of 'extremely burdensome treatment'.

If she had, for example, reached out and switched off the ventilator herself in order to end her life, such an action would be considered suicide. Would her action to cease the ventilation have been respected, or would it have been restarted in order to prevent her suicide? Was it only acceptable to turn off the ventilator if all the doctors, nurses, ethicists and lawyers agreed? Who was in control of the decision? Mrs N. was fortunate that she had not asked for the ventilation to be ceased on the grounds that she wanted to end her life because it had no quality. She would have found the going tough as such a request does not fit the sophistry required to be allowed to die with dignity in some places. Fortunately the *Medical Treatment Act* now leaves only the person concerned as the decision maker (except on occasions the psychiatrist).

If Jane's death was suicide, then was not my involvement one of assisting that suicide? I had suggested the idea to Jane, I had planned the matter with her in advance and, by providing the medication, I had allowed her to carry out her refusal of treatment in circumstances where she probably would not otherwise have been able to. I am certain that she would not have been able to withstand the physical, psychological and emotional suffering of deliberate death by dehydration without assistance.

Whilst waiting for the coroner to answer my question about the necessity to report such a death, I wrote an article that was published in *The Age*.[14] I suggested that I had assisted in that suicide, but that because of the way it occurred, within the ambience of the *Medical*

Treatment Act, it was arguably not a crime. When the coroner finally made his finding some two years later, he came to the same conclusion.

In that *Age* article, I posed the question as to why such a shameful and protracted method of assisting a suicide was legitimate, while the provision of a lethal dose of barbiturates to Jane was assumed to be illegal. With barbiturates, she could have died quietly, without fuss, in her sister's home, surrounded by her family and friends. She could have said goodbye and gone quickly to sleep, and died in less than two hours. Instead, she died by subterfuge, in a protracted manner and by hypocritical means, in a way that caused great stress and sadness for her family. There was no dignity, only futility; no honour, only shame. I had a moral responsibility for Jane's death, but the way it occurred, through lack of real choice, left me morally and emotionally distressed.

Like so many other deaths of terminally and hopelessly ill people in our society, the manner of this death was a façade to protect the outdated idea that to relieve intolerable suffering by hastening death at the request of a rational person is a crime. Why does society impose on someone like Jane an iron obligation to choose between either a life of abject suffering and despair or an undignified death?

14

PROVOKING THE CORONER

*'Because the goal of relieving pain and suffering can be attained only
by obtunding the patient until death ensues, the patient's death becomes
the end point and, therefore, one of the intended goals. Those goals do
not differ from those of physician-assisted suicide, or, for that matter,
voluntary euthanasia. Terminal sedation, we would claim, differs from
some form of active voluntary euthanasia in that it has not been, and
is unlikely to be, legally challenged.'*[1]

Professor Erich Loewy, University of California

It is most unusual to be asked to see a person in a palliative care institution who makes a request for assistance to die. People in palliative
care who make such requests are usually taken seriously by their carers,
and intense efforts are made to find out why the request is being
made and to improve the palliation. Such a request is likely to lead to
intense analysis of medical, psychological, spiritual and social issues, with
the assumption that something must have been missed for such a request
to be made. In many instances this is entirely appropriate, but in some
it can amount to duress. All the medical and psychological power of

the palliative care team is brought to bear on the weakened patient. I have seen an experienced medical practitioner, suffering from terminal prostate cancer and paraplegia from it spreading to his spine, persuaded by a palliative care specialist to undergo antibiotic and intravenous fluid management for a perforated irradiated bowel—utterly futile treatment that simply prolonged his suffering and resulted in agonising dying. It takes a particularly strong individual to insist that he is not a mental, psychological or spiritual waif who does not know his own mind.

Howard was such a man. I had known him in a slight way for some years, and had recognised him as a proud, self-sufficient and successful man who did not suffer fools gladly. At the age of seventy-nine, having lost most of his independence, he found himself in a Catholic palliative care hospice, very much against his wishes. He had developed a malignant melanoma on his back, which was excised along with related lymph glands, but the cancer recurred in his armpit, with secondary deposits in the lungs, ribs and brain. As a result of the spread to his brain, he had developed epileptic fits and then a profound permanent paralysis of his right arm and leg. He could no longer walk and was confined to bed. His elderly wife was unable to look after him in their apartment, and so he was admitted to the hospice, and would certainly remain there until he died, or was transferred to a nursing home. This he would not accept. He was dying, but the time of his death was quite uncertain, possibly not for a month or two, and certainly not imminent.

Apart from his complete dependence, he was suffering only occasional pain and some occasional mental confusion. He was being treated with a drug cocktail to relieve brain swelling, prevent fits and provide mild sedation. He accepted that his death was inevitable, but did not wish to continue living in dependence, in slow decline, and almost certainly with progressive loss of cognition and personality. This fear was realistic.

Dr Eduardo Bruera and colleagues found, in a prospective study of sixty-one consecutive patients admitted to a palliative care ward, that

83 per cent presented with cognitive failure on average sixteen days before death.[2] Howard had decided to cease eating and drinking as he found his situation intolerable. He had been refusing food and fluids for three days, but was not being given assistance with significant sedation, and it seemed he was not likely to get it in his present place of care. At this point, his wife asked me to visit him.

When I saw him, he was quite lucid and determined to end his life, and was prepared to cease drinking and eating to do so. Unlike Jane, he had come to his own conclusion to cease food and fluids, but was receiving, in his view, inadequate palliation of his resulting distress. His death was not imminent from his cancer and he would probably 'live' for up to another two months. He indicated that his discussions with the staff in the hospice gave no indication of support to make this an easy process. They apparently did not agree with the views of Professor Bernat about adequate sedation in this situation,[3] and their provision of sedatives was miserly. They were more inclined to side with philosopher Ellen McGee that 'hospice presents an ideal of continued care, of valuing the individual even when he does not value himself'.[4] There was clearly a conflict between what Howard wanted, what he saw as in his best interests, and what the palliative care team was prepared to provide. One had to wonder in whose best interests they were working, and whose autonomy they were respecting.

I told him that I fully supported his decision in the circumstances, that I believed his action was legitimate and that I could provide him with aggressive sedation that would make him sleep, to relieve any suffering he might have whilst he stopped drinking. However, I would have to transfer him to another hospital to do this, and he would have to request that transfer.

He was duly transferred to my hospital that evening and completed a Refusal of Treatment certificate, refusing treatment generally and artificial hydration specifically. He had already been refusing any intake of fluids for four days. He requested sedation and analgesics to keep him free of distress. It was clear by the next morning that his decision to refuse all food and fluids was genuine, and he could not take his oral medication without fluid. All oral medication was stopped, and replaced by midazolam (80 mg/24 hours) and morphine (40 mg/24 hours) by subcutaneous infusion to relieve pain and provide continuous sedation. Before this commenced, his family was given the opportunity to say goodbye to him. They all knew he was destined to die, and why, and accepted his choice. This medication regime was effective in making him sleep over the next thirty hours. At that time he could be wakened to establish he was comfortable. His urine output was very low, consistent with dehydration. He died peacefully after sleeping comfortably through the following thirty hours, having commenced sedation eighty-one hours previously.

On this occasion, Howard had remained essentially well sedated for the whole period, as the starting dose of sedative was better selected than for Pamela, and was essentially unchanged throughout this period. The whole process was more effective compared to Jane, and obviously quicker; this was largely serendipitous, as this man was much bigger than Jane, but he was also weaker due to his cancer, and his dehydration had a head start before I was involved. Whatever the reasons, this was an acceptable process for his family. For me, it was obviously a better managed process than that of Pamela, and emotionally less damaging compared to the protracted dying of Jane. But the essential question does not go away—why must these people have to undertake the psychologically challenging course of dehydrating themselves to death, even with the help of sedation?

Having received no advice from the coroner advising me whether such a death was reportable, I duly reported Howard's death. The report asked the question whether this was an unnatural death, possibly a suicide, and I indicated clearly that Howard had deliberately refused fluids in order to hasten his death. My provisional cause of death was dehydration due to refusal of fluids, with sedation and widespread malignant melanoma as contributory factors. The only distinctions between this process and that of Jane were that Howard reached his own conclusion to cease food and fluids, and he had a reasonably predictable end-of-life trajectory.

I had discussed the need for reporting the death with Howard and his wife. I also advised that I did not think that an autopsy would be necessary, and that his wife could object to an autopsy. To my surprise, within twenty-four hours, I had a phone call from a technician at the Coroner's Office, expressing the opinion that the death need not be reported, that it was a death due to natural causes, and asking me to sign a death certificate! I was surprised because I was still waiting, nearly three years after the event, for an official indication from the coroner as to whether the death of Pamela, in very similar circumstances, was reportable, and here I was being expected to accept the phone report of a technician as a basis for conclusion. Naturally I declined. The death certificate was quickly issued, signed by the pathologist (without any discussion with me, the treating physician). He determined that the cause of death was 'probable dehydration (on clinical grounds) and bronchopneumonia following sedation in a man with metastatic melanoma'; that is, due to 'natural causes'. The coroner's letter to Howard's wife indicated that he had finished the investigation and believed an inquest was not necessary, but I received no communication from the coroner. I eventually received a letter some months later, in response to my further request for information, stating that

> The death of [Howard] was determined not to be 'a reportable death' pursuant to the *Coroners Act 1985*. As you are aware, in many instances deaths are reported to the Coroner, but subsequently a doctor will issue a death certificate. In this case, acting on the advice of a pathologist and upon the production of a death certificate, the Coroner determined that the death was not a 'reportable death' and he did not have the jurisdiction to investigate further.

Although I had not had any official communication from the coroner until December 2000, I knew in early May that the case had been deemed 'not reportable'. The question that I first asked the coroner in 1995 had been answered, it seems reluctantly and without any formal communication. I was pleased because I felt it confirmed some important considerations. I had gone to a great deal of trouble to establish these conclusions, yet they were probably not apparent to many Victorian doctors. It seemed highly likely that the coroner, who had been unhelpful in clarifying the practical application of the *Coroners Act*, would not take any action to publicise them. I therefore called a press conference, under the auspices of the Voluntary Euthanasia Society of Victoria, and made known the details of the three cases that I had reported to the coroner, and the conclusions I had drawn. I spelt out the implications that followed from these conclusions, namely that:

Doctors now know that they can:

- aggressively sedate patients with incurable illness who refuse to eat and drink
- aggressively sedate patients who are terminally ill who refuse further treatment and request sedation to relieve pain and suffering;

and that patients and their relatives now know that they can:

- ask for aggressive relief of pain and suffering, if this is not happening, and expect an appropriate response
- refuse to eat and drink and expect any suffering so caused to be relieved.

When interviewed by *The Age*,[5] the coroner said my conclusions were inappropriate, as the case to which I was referring was not a 'reportable death' and therefore not the subject of a finding! Was he saying that this death, due to deliberate dehydration on the part of the patient, and aided by deliberate sedation by the doctor, had not, when reported to him with reference to suicide and unnatural death, been given any consideration?

It certainly had, and both the pathologist and the coroner had confirmed that the death was 'not unnatural'. I had ceased to be amazed at how the Coroner's Office was trying to avoid making any sensible or definitive statement on these issues. I wrote to the coroner requesting that he make his conclusions on the deaths of Pamela, Jane and Howard more widely known in the medical community, but he did not reply.

As a result of these coronial referrals, it was now clear that I could safely use terminal sedation to help relieve suffering in the future. However, by the time this was clear, I had become disenchanted with terminal sedation as an appropriate process. It usually required hospitalisation, when most people would prefer to die at home. I found the deliberately prolonged unconsciousness rather repugnant. There had to be a better way.

Perhaps the Coroner's Office is overworked and underfunded. It is probably not the coroner's role to educate the medical community. He very likely has enough to do without being provoked by irritating urologists with a hobby horse. It just seemed to this irritating urologist that informing doctors and the public of the legal status of refusing food and fluids, and terminal sedation, was important. It just might spare some people a lot of suffering.

In order to try to progress the matter, I wrote to the Attorney-General explaining the details of these cases. He replied that 'it would be inappropriate to comment on the details of a particular case as the one you raise, given the independence enjoyed by the judiciary' and 'the ultimate test of the legislation is a matter for the Courts'. Another brick wall! Another failure on the part of the relevant authorities to address this important question. Was I paranoid in feeling that there was a 'benign conspiracy' in place to bury any rational discussion of end-of-life treatment? Why was the use of terminal sedation such a secret, well known within palliative care, but denied to the general public?

Howard's story reveals that, good as palliative care is for most people, it is not a universal panacea for the terminally ill, and it is of little help for the chronically and hopelessly ill. Palliative Care Australia, the national body representing palliative care, has stated that it 'acknow-ledges that while pain and other symptoms can be helped, complete relief of suffering is not always possible, even with optimal palliative care'. It also acknowledges that it 'recognizes and respects the fact that some people rationally and consistently request deliberate ending of life'.[6] While Howard's physical symptoms were reasonably controlled, his paralysis could not be altered, nor his dependence and sense of loss of control. He faced an inevitable decline over some months, possibly punctuated by further physical disasters, with a loss of sense of purpose and worth.

The palliative care process is necessarily one of intrusiveness and involvement by a variety of people previously unknown to the person concerned. A crowd of people, from physicians, psychiatrists, counsel-lors, nurses, social workers to spiritual advisors, may descend on the patient, in a well-meaning attempt to improve the situation or alter a rational and consistent request for help in the deliberate ending of life. Some in palliative care have, in recent times, even taken to utilising 'dignity therapy' to deflect requests for assistance in hastening death, having belatedly realised after more than thirty years of dealing with dying patients, that 'psycho-social and existential issues may be of even greater concern to patients than pain and physical symptoms'.[7]

It needs to be understood that people with a terminal and/or hopeless illness are in a most debilitated condition, and are at the weak-est point in their lives. It is easy to persuade them that palliative care has all the answers, and to deflect a request for hastening of death. It is often claimed that people would be put under duress to end their lives by the passage of physician-assisted-dying legislation. There is an equal possibility that people will be put under duress to accept palliative care instead. Does it really show more respect for the vulnerability and dependency of the dying to coerce them to receive palliative care?

It should be recognised that all the power in this doctor–patient interface lies with the doctor(s) and the palliative care team. Patients need strong, determined and courageous advocates if they are not to be swamped by this power. For someone of Howard's proud and private personality, such intrusion can be an intolerable affront. Imagine someone with Howard's views being confronted by a palliative care professional with Ellen McGee's views. McGee accepts that Howard is 'making a choice for suicide out of a value system where this is a rational decision' but adds that:

> the philosophic stance which envisions the individual as always needing to be in control, as never being vulnerable, never a burden, and never in need of care, is in the hospice vision incomplete [and] these are the underlying values of the hospice approach to suicide. The clamour for self-determination in choosing death, for a so-called right to die, stems from a different and competing value system.[8]

Welcome to palliative care's respect for patient autonomy. You could be lucky enough to be treated by palliative care physician Derek Doyle (once a missionary surgeon in Africa) who believes that 'suffering is potentially creative'. His view of patient's attitudes is that 'for the first time, they have doubt about God's readiness to forgive, find it difficult if not impossible to articulate prayers, and rebel against what is happening yet must, at all costs, maintain an outward appearance of serenity and unshakeable faith'.[9] I fancy Howard would have had another stroke if he had been confronted by Dr Doyle with this homily.

It is not suffering in itself that some people wish to avoid. We can learn and grow through suffering, but it is surely pointless suffering that is the issue. If you believe in an afterlife, then suffering may seem to bring rewards in another place, but if you do not have such a belief, such homilies will be offensive.

Yet certainly not all palliative care providers feel this way. Dr Larry Librach has thirty years of experience in palliative care, and is the director at Toronto's Mount Sinai Hospital. He recently said:

There's a group of people who are very rational and very reasoned and who are suffering immeasurably and still want that option [of assisted suicide] and it's becoming less clear to me that we can refuse these people that option. We used to say palliative care would relieve all suffering, but that, of course was nonsense. [I've] seen too much suffering to be glib about it any more.[10]

Michael Ashby, Professor of Palliative Care at Monash University, has stated:

For many people who are dying it is not just a question of comfort or absence of physical suffering (framed in the negative) but a loss of function, independence and role which are hardest to bear. It is not the role of any health-care team to suggest that its ministrations can give meaning, purpose and dignity to a dying person's remaining life if that person feels that these are irretrievably lost, although sometimes this perception will change, either as a result of palliative care or for other reasons.[11]

Ashby's comments seem to me to clearly encompass Howard's situation—he had lost function, independence and role, and for him there was no meaning, purpose or dignity in his life. He was rational and was making a consistent request for assistance in relieving his suffering as he hastened his death by deliberate cessation of eating and drinking. Palliative Care Australia states that 'palliative care practice does not include deliberate ending of life, even if this is requested by the patient', yet it also states that it respects such rational and consistent requests. Was Howard requesting deliberate ending of life, or requesting palliation of his symptoms with sedation, or both? In other circumstances, palliative care experts have no difficulty providing terminal sedation. Peter Ravenscroft, Professor of Palliative Care at Newcastle University, has said he has no hesitation in acceding to requests for sleep, even deep sleep, when patients cannot be helped in any other way.[12]

Why then, could not the palliative care team in the hospice have reassured Howard that they would sedate him effectively, for palliation, if he decided to cease food and fluids, in order to hasten his death? Such sedation would not cause his death. After all, if he determined to cease food and fluids he must be considered a dying patient, and the *Medical Treatment Act* states that dying patients should receive maximal relief from pain and suffering. The answer may be found in an editorial in *The Lancet* by palliative care expert Janet Hardy:

> Death from malignant disease is rarely the calm, dignified process so often portrayed on stage and screen. It is commonly heralded by agitation, mental anguish and general unease and results in a well-recognised state, generally referred to as terminal restlessness. In many cases the cause is irreversible and it is usually inappropriate or impossible to determine all contributory factors. A common management strategy is sedation. Sedation is also used as a means of relieving specific symptoms (e.g. dyspnoea) in patients with advanced disease. Similarly, in the minority of patients in whom pain cannot be fully controlled by standard techniques and analgesics, sedation is occasionally used as the only means of relieving overwhelming distress.
>
> The stated justification is that there is no other means of relieving intractable distress in a dying patient, and that it is morally reprehensible to leave a patient to suffer intolerably. The concept of sedation causes considerable unease in many palliative care workers, most of whom are ardently opposed to any form of euthanasia or patient-assisted suicide. There is concern that sedation as the best means of symptom control in the dying may be underused because of fear of employing 'terminal sedation'.[13]

Howard was dying, his suffering was intolerable to him and was unrelievable. He did not have the terminal restlessness described by Hardy, but he did have the psychological suffering referred to by Ravenscroft, which would justify sedation. Such sedation would be palliative, and whilst it might possibly hasten death, its intention would be palliation, not deliberate causation of death. Moreover, there would be no need to report the matter to the coroner, and no illegality provided the appropriate refusal of treatment documents were completed.

Howard was not requesting deliberate ending of life, but wanted to hasten his own death by refusing food and fluids. He sought palliation of any suffering in the process, but as Hardy points out, many in palliative care see the palliative sedation as hastening death, and therefore morally if not legally challenging. Their moral interests are protected by providing minimal (if any) sedation, but this is not in the best interests of the patient.

Linda Emanuel, a forthright critic of euthanasia, has addressed this issue when describing 'anaesthetic coma' as a process to be offered to patients, with unrelievable pain or other symptoms, who are not imminently dying. This is a process of inducing coma with artificial provision of food and fluids and

> suitable monitoring to maintain the level of coma, preventing either anaesthesia-induced death or unwanted return to conscious-ness. While the patient may continue for days in this state before dying, the patient is not suffering ... [Anaesthetic coma may] offer a similar degree of relief from physical suffering as induced death but without the higher degree of moral questioning associated with physician-assisted suicide.[14]

I am appalled by such thinking. To suggest that patients endure days of coma when it is not their wish, nor probably that of their fami-lies, in order to preserve the moral integrity of the physician, is to put the interests of the physician before those of the patient and is against the fundamental ethics of medical practice. One might argue, incorrectly in my view, that this is the best available option under prevailing legal conditions, but not from an ethical point of view.

Whilst it may eliminate suffering, it does so in a way that ignores autonomy, imposes futile treatment and causes unnecessary suffering for the family.

It is clearly the case that terminal sedation can hasten death in some circumstances, and it is more likely to do so if it pursued vigorously. Luce and Luce indicate that:

> Opioids and benzodiazepines [sedatives] may depress ventilation significantly when given in high doses. Nevertheless, clinicians should be aware that administration of these drugs, even to the point of terminal sedation, is both ethically and legally sanctioned under the principle of double effect.[15]

Professor Erich Loewy, discussing terminal sedation, had this to say: 'Although such a practice may shorten life, I do not in any way oppose maximal sedation and analgesia for patients at this stage of life. Indeed I can see no rational or humane argument against such a practice'.[16]

The closer the timing of death to the commencement of sedation, the more likely it is that an allegation of hastening death might be made. Adopting a minimal or sluggish approach to sedation is an example of what Jonathon Glover would call 'moral distancing', allowing time and space to cloud judgement of the action.[17]

Despite the comments of Loewy, many doctors do not feel confident to provide such treatment. The following report appeared in *The Age*:

> Doctors are increasingly reluctant to do anything that could shorten a patient's life because of the threat of legal action, the Australian Medical Association said yesterday. Despite State laws that allow dying patients to refuse some medical treatment, doctors had become 'very much more circumspect' when treating dying patients, the AMA's Victorian branch president Mukesh Haikerwal said. 'I'm sorry to say it, but I am certainly seeing it (more

complaints about medical intervention) more', he said. 'We don't want anyone to say "you ended that person's life prematurely".'[18]

Some basic communication would go a long way.

This legal concern is felt not only in Victoria, but affects doctors everywhere. CS Cleeland, writing an editorial for the *Journal of the American Medical Association*,[19] said that the optimal treatment of pain requires aggressive use of controlled substances, potentially raising fears of regulatory scrutiny, or disapproval of professional colleagues. Writing in the same journal, Paul Kempen said, 'the medical profession's reluctance to provide narcotics on demand to cancer patients is multifactorial and clearly indicates physicians' fears to "assist suicides" or become otherwise liable of malpractice or drug abuse offence'.[20]

It is clear that a signal such as the preamble to the *Medical Treatment Act* does not give sufficient legal security to Victorian doctors. It requires clear statutory direction such as in the South Australian *Consent to Medical Treatment and Palliative Care Act 1995*, which states (clause 17) that a doctor

> incurs no civil or criminal liability by administering medical treatment with the intention of relieving pain and distress even though an incidental effect of the treatment is to hasten the death of the patient provided it occurs with the consent of the patient or their agent, is in good faith and in accordance with proper professional standards of palliative care.

It is unreasonable to expect doctors to accept risk in this area without clear laws to protect them.

The reluctance of palliative care to embrace the hastening of death as a way of respecting the patient's choice to be relieved of suffering is a fascinating example of tradition and dogma. It was laid down by Dame Cicely Saunders when she started palliative care in Britain in the 1960s. It is derived from an intensely religious approach to dying, and has never been seriously challenged.

Yet not all in palliative care agree with this. Experienced Victorian palliative care physician Brian McDonald acknowledges that he is bound by the Australian Medical Association's Code of Ethics, which does not support euthanasia. However, he states that this does not mean there hadn't been occasions when he believed euthanasia would be the most appropriate thing for a patient: 'I don't question the ethics at all of patients and families who request, and at times receive, euthanasia or assisted suicide. I think it comes down to an intimate relationship between the patient and the doctor'.[21]

Palliative care states repeatedly that it neither hastens death nor prolongs dying. This is of course a platitude, as such exactitude is impossible. In practice it cannot be accomplished. Philosophically, however, while prolonging death is clearly in no one's interests, why is hastening death so denigrated, unless there is a profound religious and moral conviction behind it?

The lack of formal palliative care along British lines has been argued by some as the reason for the Dutch moving in the direction of physician-assisted dying by direct injection or assisted suicide. However, in Belgium, formal palliative care along British lines has developed and penetrated medical care in a similar manner to the UK. The development of palliative care and voluntary euthanasia occurred together in Belgium, so that voluntary euthanasia has been integrated into palliative care, and palliative care physicians practice euthanasia no less than other physicians. Physician-assisted dying is now legal in Belgium (2002), and the guidelines of medical and palliative care, organisations endorsed the concept of integral palliative care, including euthanasia. Professor Jan Bernheim of the Belgian Free University indicates that the process of legalisation followed very different courses in Belgium and the Netherlands. In Belgium:

> The development of the movement for the legalisation of euthanasia was intellectually, politically and financially linked to the development of [palliative care] PC. We conclude that

euthanasia can be part and parcel of integral palliative care and that, contrary to mainstream fears, the development of PC and the process of legalisation of euthanasia can be mutually reinforcing.[22]

I personally applaud this integration as the ideal outcome for both patients and palliative care. It would ensure that patients do have access to every possible care and assistance in the dying process, and make it less likely that anyone's life would end without proper attention and scrutiny of the process. Poor euthanasia practice would be minimised and more acceptable palliative care would be the result, provided palliative care was fully open to respecting the patient's choice. Regrettably, that is a big proviso.

Much of the opposition to physician-assisted dying is about maintaining moral codes and maintaining palliative care as it is. Dr Ezekiel Emanuel, an opponent of legal change, recently wrote:

> It has become quite clear that even if legalized, these interventions (voluntary euthanasia by lethal injection or physician-assisted suicide) will assist very few of the dying, certainly less than 5 per cent of the 2.4 million Americans who die each year. If we, as a society, want to ensure a good death, then we must start focusing on hospice and palliative care to help the millions, and stop obsessing about euthanasia and physician-assisted suicide for the very few.[23]

His support of palliative care comes at the expense of the 'very few'—a mere 120 000 dying people! Is it not possible to do both? Fortunately not all in palliative care hold such views; Michael Ashby wrote, 'Palliative care is a model of care, not a moral crusade, and should not be used as a strategic weapon in social debates'.[24]

Emanuel's 120 000 dying people have been described as 'hard cases'. One might have thought that this would have given them grounds for serious consideration. Yet an Anglican Archbishop of Melbourne, Dr Keith Rayner, arguing against law reform, said:

> There are undoubted hard cases. While I understand that pain can be adequately managed in most cases, there are some cases where the physical and psychological pain is great indeed. The compassion we rightly feel for patients in this condition pulls the heart strings to be favourable to mercy killing. We know of course that hard cases make bad law, but we feel the impact of the hard cases none the less.[25]

However, like Emanuel, Dr Rayner seems to wash his hands of the problem.

At the same time, some in palliative care see legalisation of voluntary euthanasia as a threat. Dr John Zalcberg said of palliative care, 'This is intensive medicine. It is expensive medicine. I am scared that euthanasia will take this away'.[26] Palliative care Professor Ian Maddocks said, 'Legalization for voluntary euthanasia is not helpful to palliative care'.[27] Drs Zalcberg and Buchanan wrote in the *Medical Journal of Australia*: 'Good palliative care is a necessity, and we believe that the standard of palliative care is unlikely to improve if euthanasia is introduced. Furthermore pressure to provide improved palliative care in the community and within hospitals may wane were euthanasia to be legalized'.[28] This comment is actually incorrect as the experience in Oregon and the Netherlands has shown—since legalisation, palliative care has flourished.

Is palliative care concerned about competition in the area of dying patients? It should not be, because advocates of physician-assisted dying see its place as an adjunct to palliative care, treatment to consider when palliative care fails or is rejected by a patient. Some may perceive a hint of self-interest in such comments, as well as a reflection that access to physician-assisted dying for those receiving palliative care might actually be more attractive to some patients. Palliative care has fought hard to establish its turf over the past forty years and fears any move to diminish its growth. Ultimately, palliative care is an expression of the doctor–patient relationship rather than the patient–doctor relationship; that is, one in which the doctor is the master and the patient the servant, rather than the other way around—a subtle distinction, but one that is at the heart of patient autonomy. The proper expression of that autonomy means that the patient gets the palliative care that they want, not the palliative care that the doctor thinks they should have.

The circumstances surrounding the deaths of Harold (chapter 10), Pamela (chapter 12), Jane (chapter 13) and Howard all involved combinations of terminal sedation and lack of food and fluids. In all cases death was hastened but this was legitimate. Yet there were significant differences. For Harold, withdrawal of artificial provision of food and fluids at the request of his agent was accompanied by palliative sedation. For Pamela, her request for a hastened death was provided by palliative sedation with secondary lack of food and fluids. Jane and Howard both voluntarily ceased food and fluids in order to hasten death and were palliated by deep sedation. The fact remains that they died slowly (three to nine days) in a medically induced coma. The question is would they have made this choice if quick acting barbiturates could have been legally prescribed for them.

It is salient to reflect on the fact that the coroner had found that the deaths of Pamela and Howard were 'natural deaths' in the sense that they were not reportable deaths. They had both refused food and fluids and been deliberately rendered unconscious by medical treatment until they died. A natural death? Incredulous though it may seem, the State of Victoria says it is so.

Until September 2006, I remained extremely ambivalent about the process of voluntary refusal of food and fluids. At the World Right to Die Societies conference in Toronto, I met Dr Stan Terman, a Californian psychiatrist who has extensively researched this subject.[29] He points out that prior to the twentieth century, many people died in association with a lack of food and fluids—it used to be part of a natural death. He also explains that, provided there is quality nursing care directed to keeping the mouth and lips moist, there is little suffering with this process, at least for the first four days. After this, a gradual coma follows, which may be accompanied by some confusion and delirium. It is highly desirable to have the support of a doctor in this phase to provide some sedation. In countries where access to effective drugs for physician-assisted dying is difficult, this is an option available to all, and it is legal.

Further information has been published in 2007 in the PhD thesis of Dutch psychiatrist Boudewijn Chabot. He describes the process as 'auto-euthanasia'. It requires minimal or no medical help, but good nursing, particularly mouth care, is essential. There is constant accompaniment, conversation and music, with simple sedation as required. With good planning, most deaths were regarded as dignified, although prolonged (seven days or more). Chabot estimates that this process is perhaps twice as common in the Netherlands as medical euthanasia, because many of these people were frail and elderly, and did not qualify for euthanasia, or were denied it.

Is such a process dignified? This depends on the view of each individual who is confronted by end-of-life suffering. To my mind the time involved, and the existential distress associated with being forced (by lack of alternative choices) into this decision, make this an unattractive option. Intuitively, most people would reject this option as extreme, but I make these comments to inform them that the process is not as gruesome as one might imagine. There is still a dependence on others for the good care necessary to see this process through. Personally, given the option, I would always choose a reliable drug-induced death. Nevertheless, when I am no longer able to choose because of dementia, it is an effective way, in conjunction with the appropriate refusal of treatment, advance directive and enduring medical power of attorney documents, to avoid being force-fed or tube-fed into eternity.

15

FEAR OF THE FUTURE

'The rightness of an action must be judged in relation to the situation
in which it takes place.'

Professor Gab Kovacs, Monash University

'The powers of life are sensibly on the wane, sight becomes dim, hearing
dull, memory constantly enlarging its frightful blank and parting with
all we have ever seen and known, spirits evaporate, bodily debility
creeps on paralyzing every limb, and so faculty after faculty quits us,
and where then is life?'

Thomas Jefferson

Helen, an 80-year-old woman, lives alone in her own small home,
where she enjoys pottering in her garden. She can no longer play
golf or bridge, which she had enjoyed for many years, not because she
is becoming frail or losing her mental ability, but because she is losing
her sight. She is actually in excellent physical and mental health, taking
no medications, and thus has an excellent life prognosis—she may live
on for many years. Aye, there's the rub. She is questioning whether she

wants to do so. Her progressive loss of sight is threatening her ability to live independently. In short, she is facing the prospect of placement in a nursing home because it will soon be unsafe for her to live at home alone.

Helen has a daughter and two grandchildren. Her daughter is attentive, visits her regularly and helps her with household matters, things that her poor sight make difficult. But more than this, Helen had already lost the ability to enjoy television, film and theatre, and to be stimulated by books—the loss of enjoyment of her garden would be the last straw. Her sense of value as a mother and grandmother was minimal now; she felt that she was taking more than she could give.

Helen did not want to impose herself on her daughter should she become unable to cope with independent living. Despite her daughter's protestations, she felt that she would be a burden—it is her perception that matters, whether or not it is reality.

For most people brought up and educated in the Western world with Judeo-Christian values, the concept of unselfishness, or even more extremely, selflessness, is very powerful. We are taught to be considerate, to have empathy for others and to avoid doing acts that will impose unnecessarily on others. For women who have the experience of motherhood, this value is stamped even more powerfully by the need to nurture their child to the detriment of themselves. Women in particular retain this sense of nurture and unselfishness throughout life, even unto death itself. Many women, because they commonly live longer than their husbands, care for their husbands in their last weeks, months or even years with typical unselfishness. They take upon themselves the burden of care, but when their own time comes, many do not wish to pass the burden of caring for them onto their children and their families. They know only too well what it takes. The sense of being a burden can cause extreme distress and distaste to the point of depression. That sense of burden is an extraordinarily profound human emotion. For persons who have spent their entire lives being useful, having a role of significance and not being dependent on others, to be reduced to a state of dependence is more than they can bear. It is a denial of all that their life has represented, and can cause an existential distress of great magnitude.

Of course, those who have benefited from the selflessness of such a person usually have no hesitation in accepting the burden of their care, if it is at all possible, even at great cost to themselves and their families. However, no amount of love or care can deflect the sense of being a burden if that is the perception of an individual. Palliative care experts have identified one of the five critical concerns of dying persons as 'relieving others of the burden of their dying'.[1]

One should not think for one moment that the burden of caring is just a perception—it is a reality. Palliative Care Australia published *The Hardest Thing We Have Ever Done*, a research document on the social impact of caring for terminally ill people.[2] It reveals:

> Carers experience an increase in adverse health effects related to stress, a change in eating patterns leading to weight loss, and a disruption to sleeping patterns leading to carer fatigue. Carers have reduced opportunity for social and physical activities, further reducing their own physical wellbeing, which can lead to their social isolation, even to the point of becoming house-bound ...
> Carers report feelings such as guilt, fear, frustration, anger, resentment, anxiety, depression, loss of control and a sense of inadequacy.

Those who have benefited from the selfless care of a parent may well not feel that caring for their parent is a burden, and may well feel guilt if they do not respond fully and accept the burden, even though it may significantly disrupt their busy life. The carer may see this as a duty and an act of love. So it is, but the determination to provide such care, rather than listening carefully and allowing a parent space to go and to let go, can actually simply enhance suffering. Whilst the daughter may feel a moral debt to a parent that she is willing to repay, the parent may not wish the debt to be repaid in this way. In fact, the pursuit of care may create a situation of further distress. In some ways, the desire not to be a burden to family may be partly an act of altruism, a genuine act of love of the highest order.

The expression of a sense of being a burden should certainly act as a signal to assess carefully for depression. Yet Helen denied feeling depressed and did not appear to be so. Her general practitioner had known her for a long time and had explored this possibility. Her position was reasoned and carefully considered. The thought of a totally dependent life in a nursing home filled her with horror. Her diminished sight was a terrible suffering, but to lose her freedom and way of life also was just too grim to contemplate. She had personal experience of nursing home conditions, their limitations and indignities. She knew that there was a negligible likelihood of finding any meaningful relationship in such a place. She loathed the prospect of spending possibly ten or more years in these depressing and, for her, undignified and even frightening circumstances. And for what purpose? Was she obliged to stay alive in this situation for the 'benefit' of others?

She went to see her general practitioner, whom she had known and trusted for many years, to discuss ending her life before she lost the opportunity and the ability to do so without needing the physical assistance of others.

The letter to me from her very experienced general practitioner read as follows: 'This elderly woman, whom I have known for many years, has progressive and severe blindness. She is finding it very difficult to cope at home, and does not want to enter a nursing home. I am totally sympathetic to her point of view. Can you advise her?'

The necessity to enter a nursing home commonly occurs as a result of a relatively sudden deterioration in health (fracture, operation or stroke), but can also occur as the result of a steady, progressive and inevitable decline (frailty, multiple sclerosis or dementia). With this admission, whether sudden or anticipated, the change in life circumstances is dramatic. No matter how good the nursing home and its level of care, the sense of loss is enormous. Since entry is usually permanent, there is loss of home and most personal items, and potential for diminished contact with family and friends. There is loss of freedom, role and lifestyle (however already inhibited) and loss of control over daily activities. Clinical studies show that there is a feeling of loss of future and of a devalued self. There is a profound sense of being without choice, and that the admission was for the benefit of others. Such people feel that they are incarcerated in an environment they have not chosen, with others they have not chosen to live with and who are sometimes hostile and dangerous. They may live in fear and anguish and they simply have no choice over this decision.

Barbara Fiveash, in her conclusion to her study of *The Articulate Resident's Perspectives on Nursing Home Life*, stated:

> All people need freedom and choice; it is a basic need. This society uses segregation in the form of imprisonment to punish people for their crimes. Older sick and disabled people are aware that they have been segregated from the main-stream culture, and some view themselves as being imprisoned, or inmates. They are unaware, however, of what crime they have committed, except to be old and have difficulty looking after themselves.[3]

A first-hand account by a rational octogenarian on the impact of the nursing home experience is described in the story of Marion Miller in the recent publication *Seven Dying Australians*.[4] She says, 'Every day I hope that I won't wake up in the morning. I want to die'. She concludes her story: 'I never thought this would happen to me. If I'd known in time I would have done something about it. I hate to think beyond each day. And though there are worse places, the fact is that when it comes to institutional living, there is no good place. No good place'.

For many people with experience of nursing homes, the prospect of such an end to life is daunting, and I have enormous sympathy with someone who is facing such a circumstance. How much more distressing would this be for someone without sight to help them. Can you imagine the sense of dependence, not simply of being frail but also of being blind, and of moving into a strange environment? And what of the fear every time some unknown person enters one's room? Few people ever choose to enter a nursing home—they could be regarded as our 'second prison system', and entry is a 'life sentence'.

How often do we hear the phrase 'she suffered a loss'? This epitomises the fact that suffering is related to loss, in any sense or situation. Helen had already suffered the almost complete loss of sight and all the enjoyments and functions that accompany that loss. She was now facing the critical losses associated with entry to a nursing home.

Helen faced two serious dilemmas. Once she entered a nursing home she would lose virtually all privacy, and would no longer be in an environment where she would be free from the surveillance and interference that would prevent her from taking her own life. Moreover, as her vision faded, her ability to recognise medication, prepare it correctly and ingest it safely would be ebbing away. Any mistake could have disastrous effects, possibly leaving her damaged but not dead.

Although I have never worked in close association with a nursing home, I have attended, during forty years of practice, many people in nursing homes, and visited friends there. Despite the best of attention and care, these can be depressing places, particularly for the mentally competent person, since a high proportion of the inmates are cognitively impaired, usually suffering from some degree of dementia. Even where most of the severe dementia sufferers are now segregated in special dementia units, the remaining residents may at times be aggressive and sometimes dangerous. To be mentally competent in a nursing home where two out of every three residents is demented is daunting. And it is extremely hard to find companions for interesting conversation amongst the others—the remaining patients will be there because of extreme frailty, or loss of mobility as a result of osteoporosis, arthritis, hip fractures, Parkinson's disease, or chronic paralytic diseases such as severe stroke, multiple sclerosis or MND. Nursing homes are not called 'God's waiting room' for nothing.

I felt great empathy for Helen's request for my help to end her life with dignity and certainty. It seemed that she had given the matter consideration for some time, and although her request did not seem to be influenced by depression, I felt that I needed some time to get acquainted with her to make sure that she was not depressed and that she was making a persistent request. This was also potentially moving beyond the realms of the terminally ill. It was a very considerable further step in the journey.

I offered her my support in principle, asked her to think carefully and deeply about the matter, and agreed to see her again in three months if she still wanted my advice. I indicated the sort of medicine that she would need to achieve her aim. My letter to her referring doctor indicated my empathy and understanding for her situation, suggested that he assess her carefully for depression, and suggested medication that he might provide for her. I was quietly hoping she would not return.

Three months later, she did return, having obtained the medication I had suggested, and was seeking my advice and assistance in using it. She was clearly determined, yet she was relaxed, balanced and positive. I went over the issues with her, discussed her family situation, what further activities she might pursue in order to defer her decision. She could not be budged. She could see the date ahead, a time when her daughter would be away for a few days, so that she would have freedom from disturbance. She was adamant she did not want to discuss the matter with her daughter, as I had suggested. Whilst I believe it is usually desirable for the family to be involved to encourage their understanding and support, for the closure of family 'business', and an avoidance of unpleasant shocks, family dynamics do not always allow this. I don't believe that people with otherwise compelling situations should be forced to disclose their plans. There must be respect for their judgement in this as with other aspects of assisted suicide, such as autonomy and depth of suffering.

In this situation, the absence of law creates another dimension—the question of pre-emptive action to avoid the sufferer being left high and dry by a sudden change in circumstances. The need for Helen to take her life in a clandestine and secret way created specific circumstances which could easily be overrun by a sudden increase in her blindness or some other health event. The legal status quo, in a way, forced her to consider acting before the situation she wanted to avoid, the nursing home, was actually upon her. Helen was holding on by the skin of her teeth, and had no regrets at having to act perhaps a little prematurely—she was ready.

Helen's suffering was as much existential as physical. She certainly had significant blindness, much more of a burden developing later in life when helpful strategies are more difficult to employ; but fear of prolonged incarceration in a hostile, undignified environment was the driving matter. She had no physical pain—only a grinding psychological pain—a fear of being trapped for years in a situation that she felt would be repugnant to her. As Eric Cassell wrote, 'fear of the future contributes to suffering',[5] while another of the five critical concerns expressed by palliative care experts of dying persons is 'achieving control'.[6]

I could have argued that she should give the nursing home a chance, when it became necessary, and that I would help her if it proved to be as she feared. But once she was in the home, any chance of assistance would be gone. Like Jane, she would be trapped. She was therefore forced to consider pre-emptive action. In my view, the status quo created by current legislation has harsh implications that those responsible for the law are blindly unaware of.

She now needed specific advice and support. She had acquired a lethal dose of sedatives, provided by her own doctor's prescription. The cooperation of this very experienced general practitioner who had known her for many years was most reassuring, indicating that my support was also appropriate. His was a sound second opinion, in an area where second or more opinions are very important, but hard to obtain in covert practice. It is essential that one's innate sympathy for a person's suffering does not introduce bias into one's decisions.

Being blind, Helen had a need for more than the usual advice. I agreed to meet her late on the day she had chosen to end her life. I drove to her home around 5 p.m. and parked some distance away. She was really bright and cheerful when she answered the door. It always amazes me how calm and relaxed people are when they are about to end their lives—provided they have carefully considered their action and have come to terms with their mortality and accepted their death. Acceptance of the reality of death is an essential requirement to achieving a good death—it is a mark of maturity when a person facing death can make that transition. The difficulty of accepting the reality and inevitability of death is a significant reason why some people cannot come to terms with the concept of physician-assisted dying. If that transition occurs, there is a characteristic lack of fear and absence of sadness, except for the leaving of loved ones; rather, a sense of relief that they are in control and are about to escape from the severe distress and suffering which has been troubling, even engulfing them.

Proponents of palliative care speak of the importance of closure and of dealing with spiritual issues as some of the key features of a palliative care assisted death. They seem to feel that closure and spiritual matters are unaddressed in physician-assisted dying. Physician-assisted suicide is a different way of dying to a palliative care managed death— it is a less medicalised, less intrusive death that can be just as readily accompanied by acceptance and closure, and as much spiritual calm as the person desires. It is the impact of present legal circumstances that forces some people to die, regrettably, alone.

Helen offered me a drink—we shared a Scotch as we talked, and she showed me her house and her garden, and she shared some of her memories with me. Then I supervised her as she ground her tablets into a powder, and placed it in solution with some alcohol and orange juice. This was taking me to a new level of assistance in suicide where I had not gone before, but there was no alternative—her lack of sight was such that she required my help. We talked in detail and repeatedly as to how she should proceed, including taking an anti-emetic to prevent vomiting before the sedative dose. She knew her daughter would visit her when she returned home the next day, and would call her local doctor. He would not be surprised to find that she had died—of a heart attack.

After one for the road, she bade me farewell as I vanished into the darkness, sad only that she felt that she had to die alone. Any doubts about my actions were quelled by the memory of my aunt who at an advanced age suffered a severe paralytic stroke which left her completely paralysed, confined to bed in a nursing home and unable to talk. Every day when her daughter visited, her mother would grimace in an angry frustrated manner, and draw the index finger of her good hand across her throat. She had a hopeless illness, not necessarily a terminal illness, but every day in the nursing home was absolute hell from which she could not escape, except by dying. This she eventually did, some seven months later, largely by starving and dehydrating herself to death.

In 2006, a group of eminent Australian palliative care specialists found that 'The most common factors associated with a desire for hastened death appear to be: burden to others, loss of autonomy (and an associated desire to control the circumstances of death), physical symptoms (such as pain), depression and hopelessness, and existential concerns and fear of the future'.[7] Though Helen did not have depression or pain, she had all the other characteristics. My conscience was easy.

Helen's death was not imminent. She did not have a terminal illness. She had a hopeless illness. A chronic, slowly progressive illness, for which there was no treatment. Her progressive blindness, at her advanced age, created an existential suffering that was profound and increasing. Such suffering cannot be palliated, can be expected to increase, and will go on for an unpredictable but probably long time.

Ultimately it is not the illness, whether it is terminal or hopeless, that matters, but the nature of the suffering, and whether it can be effectively relieved. Thus, it is a serious mistake to exclude people with hopeless illness from the physician-assisted-dying debate. In the case of hopeless illness, however, even stricter safeguards, such as mandatory psychiatric consultation and significant cooling off periods, should be in place to prevent error.

I am sure some people will say Helen must have been depressed to have committed suicide. Let me say I do not think she committed suicide. Certainly she took her own life, but she did so only after careful and prolonged consideration, in a calm and gentle manner to prevent further harm to her person and her psyche, in order to preserve her dignity. She was one of the least depressed persons you could meet when she ended her life. I regard the word suicide as totally inappropriate in these circumstances.

The almost universal use of the word 'commit' as a qualification of suicide says it all. We 'commit murder', we 'commit manslaughter', we 'commit a felony', we 'commit infanticide'. These are all acknowledged crimes, but suicide is not a crime. The continued use of this phrase acknowledges the mindset with which we view 'suicide'.

In this book I use the term 'physician-assisted suicide' because it is the accepted and accustomed term. However, after many years of thought, I believe the use of the word 'suicide' is entirely inappropriate, even insulting, in the circumstances. Suicide has a long history, from concepts of honour, altruism and humanity in classical Greek times, to those of sin, cowardice and disgrace in the Christian era. A crime until the 1960s, it is now considered to be commonly the result of mental instability and is surrounded by stigma and shame, which makes it an inappropriate word to use in relation to both hopeless and terminal illness. Peggy Battin expressed this concisely:

> This issue is difficult for thinkers moulded by scientific and cultural attitudes insisting on the psycho-pathology and immorality of suicide. Most crucial, perhaps, is the fact that, although paternalistic and socially interested prevention of suicide is very widely practiced, the facilitation or encouragement of suicide, if it occurs at all, must take

place without social support or regulation of any kind. It is the lack of cultural regulation of the facilitation of suicide, in cases in which it may be warranted, which might be identified as the most danger-ous legacy of the suicide taboo.[8]

Today, it is a single word that covers a vast range of contexts, and the stigma which the word carries should not be borne by any of those acts, let alone the considered act of hastening one's death when afflicted by intolerable and unrelievable suffering.

The Victorian Parliamentary Committee of Inquiry into Dying with Dignity of 1985 recognised this when it declared that refusal of treatment should not be considered to be suicide. The Victorian State Coroner, in 2003, in relation to my patient who deliberately took an overdose of morphine and sedatives, found that he had 'taken his own life' and not that he had committed suicide. In 2007, the Oregon Department of Human Services also recognised the inappropriate use of the word in relation to Oregon's *Death with Dignity Act*, preferring the phrase 'Aid in Dying'. The American Academy of Hospice and Palliative Medicine accepts the occasional need for aid in dying while using the term 'Physician-assisted Death', indicating that this term 'captures the essence of the process in a more accurately descriptive fashion than the more emotionally charged designation Physician-assisted suicide'.[9] It is now time for 'suicide' to be discarded from this discussion.

It is often argued that if legislation allowed physician-assisted dying, many frail, elderly, lonely people would be persuaded by greedy relatives to end their lives prematurely, and against their will. Whilst accepting that this is a possibility, I can say that over the last fifteen years, when I have been counselling many people about their end-of-life options, I have never even once come upon this situation, and I regard the possibility as quite remote. If such a suggestion comes from the relatives rather than the individual, it should be very carefully assessed, but it would not be difficult to establish whether the sufferer fully concurred. In Oregon, medical 'Aid in Dying' has been legal for eight years, during which time 292 deaths have occurred under the Act. These deaths have been carefully analysed annually by the Oregon Health Department, and there has been no evidence of any such pressure on any occasion.

One of the commonest arguments against voluntary euthanasia is that there will inevitably be a slide towards non-voluntary euthanasia (when euthanasia has not been requested). If, as in Oregon, the law allows a doctor only to prescribe end-of-life medication but not to administer it, then control remains in the hands of the individual. Death will not occur unless the individual is totally convinced of their choice, and they are sure that the moment has come. Most people will hang on to life as long as they can, but they will know when it is time to go. Giving the person control gives them control of the time and the place. If they are not convinced, then nothing will happen. Having this control can allow the person to go forward with less anxiety, or hope-fully none. The provision of medication does not define an intention on the part of the doctor to assist—that remains perhaps the ultimate intention of the patient, but it may be an intention that is never realised. They may hang on and on, and may find that they never have the need to take any action.

This is exactly what has been found in Oregon where up to 305 of the people obtaining a prescription did not take the medication.[10] In Switzerland, where Dignitas also provides assistance with oral medication, independent analysis shows that 70 per cent of people, who have passed medical scrutiny for eligibility for provision of medication, do not proceed any further.[11] They live on without anxiety in spite of their illness or disability. It is clear that the mere fact of having control allows those patients to carry on with their lives, relieved of psycho-logical distress and anxiety, and they find a dignified death without medication. The prescription alone has had immense palliative value.

Moreover, the responsibility lies with the patient to take their own life, which is entirely appropriate. It is, after all, a huge responsibility to pass to someone else and expect them to end your life, when you can do so yourself. I do not believe that a doctor should be expected to take this responsibility unless the person making the request is completely unable to do so themselves.

It must be realised that if physician-assisted dying were legal, with the proposed safeguards (and penalties for abuse), it would occur under strict guidelines to prevent undue influence. First, there must be a request from the individual with the suffering. An initial approach may be made to a doctor by a concerned relative on behalf of a patient, but thereafter all further dialogue is with the patient, in conjunction with the relative if that is desired by the patient. Careful exploration of the origin of the request, the conviction with which it is held, and the possible influence of others must then be carried out. The doctor would have a duty under the legislation to ensure that there is no duress. This becomes a particularly important matter if the relatives appear to be involved in an intrusive manner. Second, the doctor is instructed to be sure that the patient is mentally competent to make the decision. The doctor is further instructed to be sure there is intolerable and unrelievable suffering. If this criterion does not appear to be met, the doctor should be cautious, until convinced that it is so. Moreover, the doctor must be sure that the request is persistent and enduring, allowing space for further dialogue, without the relatives if necessary. Further, the doctor can obtain a psychiatric opinion if there is any concern about mental competence. Finally, a second independent doctor must confirm all of the above requirements, and in some model legislation palliative care advice is required.

Thus, a request from relatives, or from a mentally suspect patient, will be subjected to very careful scrutiny. The request must be credible and consistent over time. The doctor will not accede to a request unless convinced about these matters.

In the Netherlands, at least 40 per cent of requests are not followed through,[12] while in Oregon only one in six requests is met. Moreover, most patients will cling to life as long as possible. I do not believe that someone can be persuaded to give up their life by another person unless they are totally convinced about doing so. If giving up life means ending it themselves, there is a very strong protection against people doing something they are not convinced they need or want to do.

Nursing homes are a relatively modern invention. In the eighteenth and nineteenth centuries we had the 'poor house' and the 'mad house'. Civility and compassion saw these disappear. In the twentieth century, families grew smaller and as a result homes grew smaller. Women developed careers and worked full-time, and the ability to care for aged parents at home diminished. People have also been living longer, acquiring all the degenerations of old age, which ultimately prevent them from continuing to care for themselves. The nursing home has been the result.

Since the relative growth of nursing homes after World War II, we now have a generation who are sixty to seventy years old who have had the experience of consigning their parents to such a place, and have memories of the grief, sadness and suffering that accompanied that process.

The renowned early twentieth-century physician Professor William Osler said, 'Pneumonia may well be called the friend of the aged. Taken off by it in an acute, short, not often painful illness, the old man escapes these cold gradations of decay, so distressing to himself and his friends'.

The growth of nursing homes was closely followed by the development of antibiotics. As a result, the old man's friend was persistently thwarted as doctors felt they were obliged to treat these infections rather than let nature take its course. Thankfully, with the rise of patient autonomy, the passage of the *Medical Treatment Act*, the increased appointment of medical agents and use of advance directives, such unwanted treatment can be avoided.

In 2004, I treated an 80-year-old man called Michael, who, because of his severe ill health and breathing difficulties, had twice tried to end his own life. On another two occasions, his probably fatal chest infection was treated without any discussion as to his right to refuse treatment. The default position of the medical profession is to treat unless someone says no. Ultimately, his daughter was granted guardianship and, after careful discussion, completed a Refusal of Treatment certificate. Thus, when Michael next developed a chest infection, he was not given antibiotics, but was treated with morphine and sedatives and slept peacefully until he died.

Kate Legge, a distinguished journalist with *The Australian*, wrote of Audrey Foyal, an elderly woman faced with unwanted incarceration in a nursing home. Audrey chose to drown herself in her daughter's swimming pool rather than undergo transportation to 'prison'.[13] Faced with ending her life in a nursing home or ending her life, she chose the latter. Not much choice considering the gruesome and painful outcome. She must have regretted the distress she knew this would cause to her family. That only serves to emphasise the enormous distress the alternative was causing her.

In my own workshops discussing end-of-life preparations, I never find a single person who is looking forward to entering a nursing home. Much of my counselling work involves talking to elderly folk living alone, whose dread is of being forced to enter a nursing home. They would prefer the choice of ending their life with dignity. As more people with experience of having placed their parents in nursing homes reach the prospect of a similar experience, the chorus of voices for another option will swell. Will their voices be heard?

16

A GOOD DEATH

Jim Dies in His Own Bed

'He prepared for his death; he died in his own bed after saying goodbye to his wife and family. It was one of those deaths that we in palliative care hope to see but rarely do.'[1]
Dr Michael Barbato, Palliative Care Specialist

'Dying is personal, and it is profound. For many, the thought of an ignoble end, steeped in decay, is abhorrent. A quiet, proud death, bodily integrity intact, is a matter of extreme consequence.'[2]
Justice Brennan, US Supreme Court, 1990; *Cruzan v. Director*

Imagine a farmer who has spent a lifetime caring for his crops and his animals. He has had his fair share of sick and dying animals that he has either put down himself or asked a veterinarian to help with. Although Jim is now seventy-nine and no longer running his own property (which has passed to one of his sons), he likes to think that he is still useful around the place. As his daughter put it, 'he continued to remain useful (in his terms) helping my brother out'. His life's work had been of a physical rather than an intellectual nature, which meant the loss of his physical ability was of significant importance to him.

Jim had shown little faith in the medical profession throughout his life, but had become a patient of mine some nine years before with prostate trouble that he could not ignore. Fortunately, he had a very effective outcome from surgery, and a secure relationship had been established between us. About a year before he died, he had experienced difficulty with swallowing, but had ignored the problem. He got by with chewing his food more than usual. Some months later the situation had deteriorated enough for his wife to persuade him to seek medical help. Over the next month or so, he saw several specialists but no firm diagnosis was made. Having a very independent streak, he always visited the specialists by himself. One specialist told him that he had a goitre (enlarged thyroid gland), which gave him a physical diagnosis and he was happy to take medication and even try acupuncture. A month or two later he was able to take a trip to England, with his wife, to visit one of his daughters. During this time it was evident that his speech was deteriorating, particularly when he was tired.

By now, Jim was concerned that something could be seriously wrong and was persuaded by his daughter, who worked in a paramedical area, to undergo further tests. However, in discussions with members of his family, he indicated that if he were seriously ill, he would refuse treatment, even if it were curative in nature.

By now, his speech and swallowing were seriously affected, so much so that he almost choked at each meal and it was impossible for him to converse because he had to concentrate so much on swallowing. Jim now agreed to further investigations and spent four days in a major Melbourne hospital, following which a diagnosis of MND was made. He was made aware that this was a fairly rapidly progressive, incurable disease that would cause an increasing sense of choking and difficulty in breathing. He was adamant that he wished to have control over his future and wanted to take his own life when the disease became intolerable. His daughter offered to contact me, as she had read of my attitudes, but not before discussing the matter with all her brothers and sisters to make sure they were in agreement with their father's decision. Jim's relief on hearing that his daughter would contact me was obvious and expressed.

On hearing his story, I agreed to visit him at his farm. I found Jim waiting anxiously in the yard as I drove up, and immediately noticed his unsteady gait as he moved to greet me, and his limp handshake in place of the usual almost crushing grip of most country men. On entering the spacious family room of the farmhouse, I was taken aback to find a gathering of family members, which increased almost by the minute as I attempted to undertake an assessment of the situation.

Such a consultation would normally take place on a one-to-one basis or with a spouse or other close family member present. The nature of such discussions is personal and the advice potentially dangerous if misunderstood or put in the wrong hands. If just one of these people was offended or unconvinced by my advice, then it would not matter what Jim thought. It could have serious implications for me. This was definitely not what I had expected, but it seemed to be what this farmer was happy with, and he did not demur at the extended family being present. I decided to go along with a general discussion of the situation, an information and educational session if you will, and see what evolved.

Jim's physical situation was as I have described. His hands were markedly weak, such that he soon would not be able to end his own life. Moreover, his ability to swallow was seriously impaired and soon the oral route might not be available. His voice was weak and tired easily, but he was still intelligible. I explained to him and his family the course of his disease without any intervention. His attitude to his predicament was also crystal clear—he wanted control; he was determined to end his life on his own terms and he did not want to linger as a shadow of his former physical self, dependent on others for his every need. He felt that he had run his race and knew that his time was near. He was balanced, rational, realistic and without a trace of depression. Some questions from the family were answered and I became increasingly confident that they would respect his decision. I explained the effect that a dose of barbiturates would have; namely, that he would quickly go to sleep and probably die within half an hour.

Further questions were dealt with as I approached the crunch. I had brought the necessary medication with me as I felt that he would need to have it now, because his situation could deteriorate suddenly and, since he was in the country, I could not guarantee to get the medication to him in time. Would I ask the family to leave us whilst I gave him the medicine together with explicit instructions as to how to take it, thereby creating an impression of distrust and emphasising the illegal nature of the act, or keep them all involved and comfortable with the naturalness of the event?

I was becoming more and more frustrated with the clandestine nature of my work in assisting people to die with dignity and was approaching the point where I would almost welcome the opportunity to defend my actions if such a challenge came to pass.

In some ways, this might not be the perfect case to defend—no second opinion, no psychiatric opinion, no prolonged treatment association or persistent request. However, I felt that this family was on the farmer's, and my, side and that I could count on their support. So I produced the medication from my pocket, described in detail how to take it, wished him well, and left.

This clinical association was brief, not what is advocated, nor what I would advocate, for legalised physician-assisted dying practice. However, I knew from my earlier talk with his daughter that he had been convinced in his mind for some time—this was not a spur of the moment decision. In even a short time, it is possible to assess the extreme state of distress of someone suffering with an advanced chronic or progressive neurological disease. It was clearly advanced, hopeless and there was no useful medical intervention. Sometimes, delay will be incredibly unkind and may lead to loss of opportunity. If I had been close by, I would have arranged to visit Jim again over the next two days but, again, the nature of clandestine practice made it difficult to do that. Had I had the slightest doubt about the correct course of action, I would have arranged another visit, but I had no doubt.

What happened next is best left to his daughter's description of events:

> I can't explain how thrilled my father was to have control of his life again and how much it meant to him.
>
> My father's condition was deteriorating. He was getting to the stage that he almost required help to eat because the muscles in his hands and arms were becoming paralysed. In addition he had a great deal of coughing because he had difficulty swallowing his saliva.
>
> During breakfast one morning he had great difficulty getting the spoon to his mouth. This was when he decided to end his life. He mentioned to my brother that he would take the barbiturate while my mother was shopping. As a family we thought that our mother would rather be present when dad took the drug. We are all pleased to think that we informed mum of our father's decision. My father was trying to do the right thing by my mother. By choice, four family members were present when dad took the medication. It was a very special time and something I won't forget. Although there were a few heated moments because a couple of family members couldn't come to terms with the finality, it is behind us now and they soon realized the importance of his decision. They thought he was ending his life far too early which I kept reminding them that the decision was entirely up to Dad alone despite what anyone else thought.
>
> When my father took the barbiturate we had encouraged him to sit on the bed and we made light of the fact he should empty his bladder beforehand. Once he took the drug he slumped into a deep sleep but was actually dead within five minutes. The whole

thing was very peaceful and he looked very relaxed and didn't appear to suffer. He was happy to the end.

Looking back on the day Dad ended his life, I can only say I have very happy feelings. Although there was mixed emotions at the time, I believe our memory of Dad's death is a lot easier to reflect on than if he'd progressed further with the illness.

There is no doubt that I assisted Jim to end his life. I advised him about medication and how to use it, and I provided it for him. On the face of things, this would appear likely to be regarded as illegal—as aiding and abetting suicide. Why would I do this? Because he made a rational and compelling request for assistance—he was facing rapidly progressive paralysis with not only the inability to swallow, but the likelihood of choking on his food and saliva. He wanted control over his future to prevent fear and depression from overwhelming what remained of his life. His response to gaining that control is clearly stated in his daughter's letter. I would argue that my assistance had therapeutic value.

What impresses me greatly about this man's story, and his family's reaction to his decision and death, is the great maturity behind it. There is no recrimination, no anger, no guilt, no embarrassment or self-delusion. The principal characteristic is acceptance of reality and of death, and an elimination of those emotions that are destructive. There is a focus on positive things, good communication, humour and sharing of emotion and adversity. This man's death is notable for its fine closure, which has left behind good memories, of peace, calm and fulfilment. It is through such fine communication that people can ease the grief of those left behind. His family is left with warm memories of his dying because of the way he handled it.

Some in palliative care make much of the importance of closure, and assume this is not possible with physician-assisted dying. This is nonsense, as this story shows. In many ways, good closure may be more readily achieved with legal physician-assisted dying. The moment of death is controlled. Closure may be planned and farewells made. These

are things that may be difficult if death is crept upon by gradual sedation. Dr Michael Barbato's comment at the head of this chapter puts
the reality of palliative care experience into perspective.

There is no doubt that dying can be hard, tough and grievous for
both families and the individual. Without good communication and
acceptance, death can be an extremely difficult time for families. It arises
from a natural sense of not wanting to lose a loved one, and from an
inability to let them go. It arises from false hope, and from trying to
maintain hope when giving permission to let go is needed. It derives
from a failure to recognise and understand suffering in general and that
of their loved one in particular. Unfortunately, it imposes an obligation and a duress to continue living, which can amount to unperceived
persecution. But as this story shows, much of that grief can be assuaged
by acceptance of dying and with excellent communication that can flow
from that acceptance. Acceptance opens the door to communication,
and allows the time remaining to be used positively. It is precious time.
If there is no acceptance and openness, you cannot say to a loved one
'when you are gone, I will miss you enormously' or 'my love for you
will not die with you'. Such poignant remarks will bring sadness, but
also joy; joy to reflect on in later years. The last phase of a dying
person's life should be celebrated, not regretted. If one is confident that
that dying phase will not be scarred by uncontrolled suffering, then it
is possible for it to be positive.

The last weeks or days of a person's life are some of the most
precious, because so little remains. They should not be crushed by
toxic anxiety. They should be liberated from fear by the confidence
of control.

Thus, Jim had the maturity, or psycho-emotional strength, to
question medical control over the end of his life, and to assert
control himself. He had the maturity to accept the reality of his
imminent dying, and the maturity to communicate his feelings to
his family about his necessity to exert his own control. It is not everybody's wish to have such control, but in a humane and pluralistic

society, it is essential that people like Jim be free to make and implement their own decisions.

Several years later, a neurologist whom I knew well referred a man in his sixties with the following simple referral letter:

> Thank you very much for seeing this most unfortunate man with mainly bulbar onset (affecting swallowing, speech and breathing), but also to a smaller extent limb, of motor neurone disease. He is intelligent and well informed, doing his own internet searches of the condition, and also watched a close friend die of the condition not so long ago.

He had no urinary symptoms, and it was obvious that the referral was to discuss aid in dying. Tragically, Victor had been married for only five months, and had probably less than two years to live. If he had been searching the internet thoroughly, he would have been aware of the research of Linda Ganzini into the attitudes of patients with MND. She found that 56 per cent of these patients would consider assisted suicide, and 44 per cent of the 56 per cent agreed with the statement 'if assisted suicide were legal, I would request a lethal prescription from a physician'. Ninety-one per cent thought the disease caused stress for family members and 65 per cent felt they were a burden. 'Although there was no difference in the prevalence of depression between patients who would consider taking a lethal dose of medication and those who would not, patients who would consider assisted suicide had higher scores for hopelessness. Hopelessness and depression were not synonymous.'[3]

Victor was indeed seeking control over the end of his life. He understood his future and wanted no part of tube feeding. I had no hesitation in providing him with advice and medication. At the end, Victor did accept PEG feeding for a few months in order to go as far as he could, and to provide a pathway for his medication when he could no longer swallow. He was clear that the provision of my advice and medication had allowed him to go further in his life with a measure of peace that would have been impossible without it.

Victor is an example of the uncommon situation where there may be a necessity for voluntary euthanasia by direct lethal injection as the only way in which an individual can end intolerable suffering and die with dignity. Once a person has lost the ability to swallow or digest oral medication, then they are unable to end their own life, even with extensive assistance from others—unless a stomach tube is placed. A person who is severely or totally paralysed but can still imbibe medication to end their life will require extensive assistance to prepare the medication in a fluid form, and physical assistance in drinking it. The German neurologist Martin Klein agrees with this concept, arguing that voluntary euthanasia by lethal injection should only be allowed if self-administration is impossible.[4] He writes:

> [this] limitation seems reasonable and necessary because physician assisted suicide cannot occur without the patient's participation, misuse is then less likely. Very seldom physician-assisted suicide might be no option, for example due to physical weakness; it is important that the patient is able to exercise the utmost control concerning his or her fate whenever possible, which should be possible in the majority of cases.

Linda Ganzini's survey of the attitudes of MND sufferers was carried out in Washington State and in Oregon, where physician-assisted suicide was legal. The decriminalisation of physician-assisted suicide in Oregon has now been thoroughly analysed over nine years of practice.[5] Careful analysis, by the Oregon Department of Human Services, of those utilising physician-assisted suicide in Oregon over six years reveals that about 90 per cent were high school or college graduates (compared to 75 per cent of the general population with similar diseases) and that about 85 per cent of such patients were receiving hospice care when they ended their lives.

It has acted as a laboratory for testing the safety of physician-assisted dying and has passed all tests, despite the dire predictions of its initial opponents. One of those, the conservative religious critic, Daniel Lee, made the following comments in 2003:

> The Oregon *Death with Dignity Act* specifies an elaborate procedure consistent with the most rigorous standards of voluntariness … It is significant that the Oregon experience to date in no way suggests that a slide down a slippery slope is imminent … When all things are considered, the arguments in favor of continued prohibition of physician-assisted suicide are not particularly compelling.

To his immense credit, he concluded his essay with these words:

> Those of us opposed to physician-assisted suicide would do well to focus our efforts on helping others discover the meaning and hope that are possible in life, even in the midst of suffering. We can accomplish far more by reaching out in a loving, caring manner to those experiencing great suffering, instead of sitting around moralizing about what they should do or not do and threatening physicians with legal penalties if they act in ways at odds with values we hold dear. If we were to do a better job of responding to suffering individuals in a loving, caring manner, physician-assisted suicide would in all likelihood be an option rarely, if ever, chosen.[6]

I totally agree with his sentiment, though not with his conclusion.

Daniel Lee's statement does him great credit because it is so ethical. Objections to physician-assisted dying are of two kinds—moral (usually based on a religious conviction) and practical (based on presumed dangers). Many who object on moral grounds base their arguments on practical objections and barely, if at all, mention their moral attitudes. Lee has strong moral objections based on religious values. He admits this and acknowledges that the practical objections are insignificant. Quite properly, he argues for better moral persuasion and better application of his moral principles.

Contrast Jim's death with that of a much younger man in a Catholic palliative care institution. He had developed MND, become totally dependent and had reached a stage where he was struggling both to swallow his own saliva and to breathe. He had reached the end of his tether and said so. He was given minimal and ineffective sedation, which increased only after a week, when his friend, the executive officer of the Voluntary Euthanasia Society of Victoria, advocated vigorously on his behalf for more palliation. He died after twelve days of profound suffering, twelve days after he was ready to go.

MND is one of those conditions that creates suffering of such a degree that Palliative Care Australia admits it cannot relieve all the suffering and distress that occurs, despite optimal palliative care. It can do so with terminal sedation, but its policy statement does not say so. Palliative care is very coy about mentioning terminal sedation.

What palliative care does for people whose suffering it cannot relieve is 'accompany' them, showing compassion and non-abandonment. This is fine—it shows sympathy, but does it show real empathy? Is it enough?

MND highlights the palliative care dilemma better than almost any other disease. Dying from this disease without medical care is an appalling experience. Dying from this disease with physician-assisted suicide (or direct injection voluntary euthanasia) can be a peaceful and positive experience. Dying from this disease with palliative care will vary from pole to pole according to the aggression of the medical intervention—essentially to the extent that death is hastened. Yet Palliative Care Australia states that it is opposed to the deliberate ending of life on request. Clearly, this leads to variable degrees of inadequate palliation in order to preserve the declared interests of palliative care, rather than respecting the autonomy of the patient. If the palliation is to be better, then the sedation must be more aggressive, but as the sedation becomes more aggressive, so does the prospect of hastening death. No doubt, those aggressive palliative care practitioners will say they are merely palliating the suffering, but they are doing more than that, and that is why conservative palliative care practitioners drag the chain. There are clear differences of opinion within palliative care on this issue.

An experienced palliative care nurse was appalled at the lack of palliation of a fellow nurse with breast cancer in a religious hospice, and received the following letter from a nun, a friend of hers who worked in that hospice: 'I am sorry that Helen's death devastated you so much. It was a shocker and none, especially her, deserved to die like that. It was so unfortunate that Ron and Meg weren't around that weekend'. It was clear that Ron and Meg were regular staff with a more liberal attitude than those who were 'caring' at the time.

These concerns about hastening death are based on certain religious and moral values rather than the medical ethics of the situation. Relief of suffering should not be only in sufficient measure as to satisfy the carers rather than the patient.

It is this predicament that led, I believe, to the Editorial in *The Lancet* by Janet Hardy, in which she said:

> The concept of sedation causes considerable unease in many palliative care workers, most of whom are ardently opposed to any form of euthanasia or patient-assisted suicide. There is concern that sedation as the best means of symptom control in the dying patient may be underused because of fear of employing 'terminal sedation'.[7]

Her admonition (echoed by others in recent times) was clearly directed at palliative care workers who were allowing their religious beliefs to conflict with the best interests of their patients. They were clearly able to see the close association of terminal sedation to voluntary euthanasia and were troubled by it, so much so that they chose either not to employ it or to do so in such an ineffectual and infrequent manner as to harm their patient.

The Australian Medical Association (AMA) Code of Ethics (1992) is relevant to this situation: 'Do not deny treatment to any patient on the basis of colour, race, religion, political beliefs or nature of illness. When a personal moral judgment or religious conscience alone prevents the recommendation of some form of therapy, inform your patient so they may seek alternative care'.

There is no doubt that religious views influence attitudes to physician-assisted dying. Many studies confirm this.[8] They undoubtedly have been influential in palliative care's position. Yet the AMA Code of Ethics suggests that patients receiving palliative care should be made aware of this position, which means not simply stating that palliative care does not endorse hastening of death, but stating why.

Does money have an influence on end-of-life decisions? Does the ability to pay influence the availability of physician-assisted dying? I can speak only for myself in saying that I have never charged for services relating to voluntary euthanasia, apart from standard fees for occasional formal consultations. I did not charge Jim, Victor, Howard or Susan. To my mind, it is a privilege to be in a position to render to a patient, as Dr Aycke Smook, a Dutch cancer surgeon, put it, 'the last treatment I can give you'. I have never been aware of a 'market' for this service. No one has ever contacted me to see what I charged because they could not afford another doctor's fees. Fortunately, it seems that those doctors who do provide assistance also see it as a privilege, and a duty. Nevertheless, in the days of criminal abortion, before Justice Menhennitt's liberalising decision,[9] there was an appalling two-tier system—clean, safe, medical abortion for those who could afford it, and dirty, dangerous 'back-yard' abortions for those who could not. There may be an analogous situation today regarding physician-assisted dying, it being available for those with knowledge and connections (rather than money), with the others taking their chance on whatever is available to them.

17

THE SUFFERING MIND

*'Depression is the most painful illness known to man, equalling or
exceeding even the most exquisite physical agony.'*
Dr John Cade, eminent Melbourne psychiatrist (discoverer of lithium
in the treatment of manic depression)

During 2003, a young university student from Sydney called Wasim
contacted me seeking advice about drugs to end his life. He had
attended a debate at Sydney University between Philip Nitschke and
theologians, and attempted to obtain drugs from Philip, but his request
was properly declined. Thwarted in that direction, he came to
Melbourne for assistance. When I talked to him, he told me that his
family had relatively recently migrated to Australia from the Middle
East, and he was having some serious conflict over traditional family
and religious values and saw his parents' discipline as harsh. He had
dropped out of his university course and left home. He had not told
his parents he had come to Melbourne. It did not take long to establish
that Wasim was seriously depressed and that his request was irrational.
However, it did take nearly an hour of counselling to persuade him

that he should seek expert medical help to resolve his problems rather than taking his life. Ultimately he agreed to accompany me to the nearest public hospital emergency department for psychiatric assessment. There I spent two hours calming and reassuring him until the psychiatric assessment team could deal with him. He was admitted and treated for his psychiatric distress.

I would like to think I had done something to save Wasim's young life, and that gives me far more satisfaction than helping someone to die. Through being a doctor who is prepared to talk about dying, instead of helping Wasim to die I helped him to live. If we encourage people to talk about dying, and encourage doctors to respond in a protected environment, as many lives might be saved as are currently being lost through lack of communication. In the present circumstances, many doctors choke off such conversations through fear of getting into deep and unprotected water.

If information were available on the internet regarding a readily prepared cocktail of chemicals to end life reliably, I believe Wasim was smart enough to find it and possibly become a 'suicide' statistic. This is why I am totally opposed to the development of a 'peaceful pill', a 'make it yourself' recipe that would inevitably escape into public knowledge and websites and, without the influence of any medical assessment or advice, become a pathway to disaster. There is a great risk that the availability of do-it-yourself euthanasia, using methods being developed by Dr Philip Nitschke, will become widespread. Since such methods do not require the advice or counselling of a doctor, their use will almost certainly spread beyond those people who have a terminal and/or hopeless illness to people with temporary psychological disturbances or to people whose wish to die would evaporate with help and change of circumstances. While the development of drugs that could allow this, with certainty and dignity, will be very difficult, Dr Nitschke has already developed a gaseous method that seems to be simple and effective, and perhaps a chemical method. If government does not move quickly to address this issue of physician-assisted dying, then carte blanche 'suicide' will be a reality, and there will be no possible means of control. There may be no going back.

That is why I believe there must be safeguards, and a framework for medical advice, for anyone considering ending their life because of intolerable suffering. This approach places me in conflict with Philip Nitschke and many other older people who want control over their lives without having to go through medical hoops to justify their decision. To me, it would be a Pyrrhic victory if euthanasia became a legal reality and even a small number of people died prematurely without due consideration because of a lack of rigorous safeguards.

I arrived home late in the evening to find three recorded messages on my phone. Their tone was urgent and tense, frantic and hopeful. It was not long after the death of Nancy Crick in May 2002, so widely pub-licised by Philip Nitschke, during which time I had been very active in the media debate supporting the principle of physician-assisted dying in specific circumstances. The calls were from Frank, who told me he suffered from paranoid schizophrenia and wanted advice as to how he could end his life effectively. He heard voices telling him to tattoo his face with the words 'I hate my mother', and he had twice tried to end his life.

What a dilemma. I had no experience in psychiatry but had known friends who had suffered from severe depression. I had recently read Andrew Solomon's classic *The Noonday Demon* about his own and others' battles with depression.[1] It is no wonder John Cade made the statement that heads this chapter. Thus I was sensitive to the severe mental suffering this man may have had, but unsure how I could assess his mental ability to make a rational decision, the backbone of any med-ical assistance in dying. Should I have ignored his calls? Eventually, he would speak to me—would I abruptly tell him I could not help him and hang up? I rang him.

He told me his story and I kept him talking, learning more about him and indicating my concern. I finally told him I could not think of helping him without an indication from his psychiatrist that he was rational and able to make sound decisions. I anticipated this would not be the case.

A week later, I received a letter from Frank's psychiatrist and a number of phone calls from Frank. The letter said, 'It is my clinical opinion that Frank is capable of making informed rational decisions about treatment for his psychiatric illness'. Reassuring as this was, that Frank had rational moments when he could weigh decisions, it did not necessarily mean he was competent to make the ultimate decision. What now, Frank asked? Indeed! I agreed to meet him in my office.

He was in his mid-thirties and appeared quite calm. He told me that he had been treated for paranoid schizophrenia for about three and a half years. His problem was hearing voices, principally those of Mark Hughes and the devil. They made him set fire to his couch, and they made him vomit. They were now telling him to tattoo his forehead.

He had been treated by a number of consultant psychiatrists with many different anti-psychotic medications and he seemed to take his medication consistently (a failure in many schizophrenics). He had, in fact, just been released from in-patient care to adjust his medication, but he said the change had made no difference to his voices. He had previously had electro-convulsive therapy but with no effect.

He was not married, but had regular contact with his mother and brother. He was a skilled tradesman but was unable to work. He had contemplated taking his own life for more than twelve months, and had considered hanging himself and jumping in front of a train. The 'devil' was telling him to end his life; he had already tried to gas himself using his car exhaust, and on another occasion six months ago, he had taken all his medication and ended up in intensive care.

He was convinced he would eventually succumb to the voices and get his forehead tattooed, and then he would become a social outcast. He was equally sure he would take his life if this happened, and he wanted to do this with security, some dignity and without involving and shocking others.

There is no doubt this man had enormous mental torment. One should not fail to understand that when a mentally disturbed person attempts to take his own life, it is a rational decision to them; such is the depth of their mental anguish from which they can see no escape. It is society that sees their action as irrational, which it is in the broader sense, if they do have a temporary, treatable illness. But it may be only in retrospect that this judgement can be made. The important question to me was: could further changes to treatment be made that would alter Frank's present state of mind? If they could, then I had no business assisting him to end his life.

I told him he should be patient and continue treatment to its maximum efficiency. He had indicated he did not want to die, but was afraid he would not be able to resist the voices. I promised him I would talk with his psychiatrist, impressing on her his suicidal state and the lack of effect of current therapy. I subsequently had a long conversation with her, during which she confirmed Frank's diagnosis and history, the difficulties of treatment and his poor response, but indicated there was further scope for an increase in his drug therapy. We agreed I should support him in therapy. Finally, after a torrent of further messages from Frank, I called him and gave him that advice. He told me he would continue to try to find a source of Nembutal through the internet. I did not hear from him again, despite attempting contact on a number of occasions through the phone number he had given me.

Nembutal is the proprietary name for the quick-acting barbiturate pentobarbital, which is the barbiturate of choice for a dignified end of life. Unfortunately, it is no longer available on a doctor's prescription, but is available to veterinarians. It is difficult to obtain, though anecdote indicates that it can be obtained in Mexico. Internet sources are not recommended. Dr Philip Nitschke is attempting to develop ways in which people might make this drug for themselves. So far, these attempts have been, not surprisingly, unsuccessful. Although pentobarbital is not a complex chemical, producing it as a clean chemical with reliable purity and strength is a sophisticated manufacturing exercise.

Of more concern is the prospect of such information being placed on websites where uncontrolled public access is possible. I regard this as dangerous and extremely irresponsible. I am strongly opposed to such activity.

In one sense I felt relieved at this outcome, because I no longer had the feeling of responsibility of assisting him to make his decision. In another sense, I felt sad, because I had a very strong feeling the outcome was predictable no matter what anyone did, and this was a human tragedy of Shakespearean proportions. I also felt guilty, because this inevitability made me feel that his further suffering whilst he tried to find a humane solution was probably avoidable, and perhaps I was ducking the issue. The reality is that it is not possible to solve, or even begin to solve, everybody's problems. Finally, there was again anger that society had so little recognition of the intense nature of mental suffering, and that the government and the community gave so little consideration to the provision of adequate services to the mentally ill.

Whilst trying to resolve whether I should help Frank, I read Anne Deveson's outstanding book, *Tell Me I'm Here*,[2] which discusses schizophrenia in the context of her son's illness. This harrowing story details the terrible lack of support for these patients and their families, and impressed me with how complicated and variable this illness was. Up to 25 per cent of people with schizophrenia take their own lives, often after many repeated but unsuccessful or thwarted attempts. These are not simple 'cries for help' (as some would say of 'suicide' attempts), but a reflection of deep mental anguish. Some chronic schizophrenia and some chronic depression can be essentially unresponsive to treatment. For some, it is truly a hopeless illness.

Is there not a place in these circumstances, where further 'suicide' attempts are certain, to consider a request for assistance in dying in order to prevent a violent end or, at least, non-interference with the process if that is the considered decision of the sufferer, taken at a time of informed rationality?

The Swiss Federal Court has acknowledged, as a guaranteed European human right, that a person may determine the manner and time of his or her end of life. The court basically granted the mentally ill this same right, provided they have capacity for discernment. The Dutch courts have made the same declaration. To deny decision-making capacity to a schizophrenic in remission, and therefore rational, is the ultimate discriminatory act against the disabled and vulnerable. I have spoken to a number of psychiatrists who would agree.

We should also not forget the tragic impact of violent 'suicides' on innocent bystanders—on the driver of a train or car who may become the instrument of a 'suicide', and on those who discover the body and may have to clean up the scene. The loved ones may be scarred forever by the gruesome circumstances in which 'suicide' can occur.

Ultimately, I believe I made the right decision not to help Frank. I simply do not have the necessary expertise to make such decisions, and it would require sustained treatment by psychiatrists before such a decision should be considered. Much as I wanted to help him with his suffering, emotion alone is not a basis for such decisions. This is another reason why such decisions need second or more opinions from appropriately trained doctors. The second opinion from Frank's psychiatrist helped me to make the correct decision, but in the present legal climate where covert euthanasia is the norm, second opinions are not the norm, and much harm may ensue from this. Over the past ten years, I have had many requests for assistance in dying from people whose approach, demeanour and story strongly suggested significant emotional or mental instability, unrelated to any apparently serious physical illness. I have always urged them to seek further professional help, though sometimes reluctantly, because many had already done that extensively and found it wanting.

The Netherlands voluntary euthanasia legislation, passed in 2001 after more than twenty-five years of careful debate, clinical study and legal test cases, determined that the principal criterion for euthanasia was that 'the patient's suffering was lasting and unbearable'. This description does not exclude physician-assisted dying for a patient with mental illness, but the requirements of due care call for two 'second' opinions, including that of at least one psychiatrist, and very careful consideration of the possibility of diminished decision-making capacity. This position was largely reached following the trial in the Dutch Supreme Court of psychiatrist Dr Boudewijn Chabot, who assisted the death of his patient who suffered from an adjustment disorder consisting of a depressed mood, without psychotic signs, in the context of a complicated bereavement process. In Chabot's opinion, supported by seven colleagues, his patient was experiencing intense, long-term psychic suffering that was unbearable and without prospect of improvement. Chabot was found technically guilty (but not punished) because none of the seven experts that he consulted personally saw his patient (none of them considered it necessary to examine her, and the court rightly criticised this). However, the principle of psychic suffering being grounds of necessity for physician-assisted dying is established. However, if psychiatric illness is the principal concern, I would recommend that at least two psychiatrists provide an opinion.

The question of depression is very important in the debate about assisted dying. Margaret (chapter 8) was admitted to palliative care late in the course of her illness for the treatment of presumed depression. She found the suggestion insulting. There is no doubt that depression can be a serious reality for people faced with imminent and certain death, particularly when it is accompanied by severe physical symptoms or loss of function. To be threatened by complete paralysis, permanent hospitalisation, followed by loss of the ability to speak and swallow (with the threat of a stomach tube for feeding) and then slow loss of the ability to breathe, would suffice to alter anyone's mood. The joy of life would leave most people to be replaced by a depressed mood, but this is a reaction to particular physical circumstances that cannot be altered. Though some people can transcend severe suffering and find

meaning in their lives, others are not to be judged if they do not. It
is not remarkable that someone would have a depressed mood in these
circumstances—it would be more remarkable if they did not! However,
there is a significant difference between a depressed mood in response
to adverse circumstances and clinical depression due solely to psychological causes.

Mary Jane Massie and associates discussed depression in terminal
illness in these terms:

> The more narrowly the term is defined, the lower the prevalence
> of depression that is reported. Depression is challenging to study
> because depressive symptoms occur on a spectrum that ranges
> from sadness to major affective disorder, and mood change may
> be difficult to evaluate when a patient is confronted by a major
> threat to life ... The diagnosis of depression in physically healthy
> patients depends heavily on the presence of somatic symptoms
> of anorexia, fatigue, insomnia, and weight loss. These indicators
> are of little value as diagnostic criteria for depression in cancer
> patients, as they are common to both cancer and depression. In
> cancer patients the diagnosis of depression must depend on
> psychologic, not somatic symptoms. These psychologic symptoms
> are dysphoric mood, feelings of helplessness, loss of self-esteem,
> feelings of worthlessness or guilt, anhedonia and thoughts of
> 'wishing for death' or 'suicide' ... Suicidal ideation requires
> careful assessment to determine whether the patient has a depres-
> sive illness, or is expressing a wish to have ultimate control over
> intolerable symptoms.[3]

Readers may consider the psychiatrist's opinion of Jane (chapter 13)
and of Susan (chapter 18). The diagnosis of depression is not exact—
it is a syndrome of symptoms and signs, many of which overlap with
symptoms that are very common in terminal illness without depression, such as loss of appetite, loss of energy, sleeplessness and loss of

hope, together with a desire to end one's life (suicidal thoughts). Some psychiatrists who deal with the terminally ill find that a very high percentage of their patients have depression. Of course, labelling a patient with a psychiatric illness can also be a convenient way to deny a request for assistance in dying. The Professor of Palliative Care at Melbourne University, psychiatrist David Kissane, has even gone to the lengths of describing his own syndrome of 'demoralisation' into which to fit these dissident patients who choose to die. He can see no circumstance whatsoever in which voluntary euthanasia is appropriate.

On the other hand, Dr Nisha Shah found, in a survey of British psychiatrists' attitudes to euthanasia, that 86 per cent thought that 'suicide' could be rational in the context of terminal illness.[4] Palliative Care Australia accepts that patients may rationally and persistently request a hastened death. Thus, while it is always possible for a patient requesting assistance in suicide to be depressed, and this possibility should be considered, many patients will still be rational.

To my mind, the relationship between the stage of the disease, the extent of physical suffering that is obvious, and the apparent degree of depression is all important. A patient who, having few if any symptoms, has just been made aware of the diagnosis of incurable cancer and requests a hastened death, is very likely to be acutely depressed; whereas a patient with only a week to live and who is in severe pain is less likely to have depression, or a treatable depression. Max Chochinov approached this problem by asking the simple question, 'Do you feel depressed?' and the answer correlated very well with the detailed psychiatric assessment.[5] Margaret was clearly answering 'no' to this question. Overlying the question of whether a particular patient is depressed or not is the question of whether treatment might be effective. It should be realised that antidepressant medication will take all of three weeks to be effective, and thus it is pointless attempting such drug therapy in a patient whose death is imminent. Moreover, the success of medication in a patient with severe unrelieved physical symptoms is low—you cannot expect that someone with symptoms of severe pain, severe breathlessness, cachexia or paralysed limbs will respond to antidepressant treatment, although you might try if there is time and the patient agrees. There should be no medical duress to undergo treatment. It no longer surprises me to find that many people requesting assistance in dying are already taking what should be effective antidepressive medication (such as Alice, Mrs Knight, Pamela and Keith).

Let me make this point very clearly. I do not advocate medical assistance in dying for anyone who is suffering from psychiatric illness. As the first story in this chapter illustrates, these people need urgent expert care. But there are some people with a chronic and/or recurrent psychiatric illness that is resistant to treatment. While it may be controlled to varying degrees, it cannot be cured. The suffering that these people endure may be no less intolerable than those with severe physical illness—it may be worse, as John Cade asserts. Because we cannot see their disability does not mean it does not exist. They deserve our consideration. Making such assessments is a matter of high skill and the province of a panel of psychiatric experts, and should be done only after the apparent failure of prolonged, sustained and intensive treatment. There needs to be the utmost restraint, but the possibility should not be denied.

18

REGAINING CONTROL

'To be, or not to be—that is the question;
Whether 'tis nobler in the mind to suffer
The slings and arrows of outrageous fortune,
Or to take arms against a sea of troubles,
And by opposing end them?'
Hamlet (*Hamlet, Prince of Denmark*, William Shakespeare)

In 2003, Susan made her own appointment to see me, without referral, but at the suggestion of her palliative care physician. She had been
suffering from a slowly growing brain tumour for eight years. She was
now thirty-two, and although the tumour growth had been halted by
radiotherapy, it was now starting to grow again. Susan had frequent head
pain, poorly controlled by medication, which caused severe side-effects.
She was now suffering severe anxiety about her future and could obtain
no answers from her carers. I arranged for her to see her psychiatrist
who reported to me as follows:

> Susan consulted me yesterday and explained that specialists
> frequently refer to her as being depressed and ascribe many of her
> physical symptoms to this. She does not believe she is depressed
> and feels that depression is being used inappropriately to explain
> her fatigue etc.
>
> I have known Susan for two years. In that time I have seen
> her go through the distress of having recurrence of her brain
> tumour and the subsequent decline of her physical health. She

224

has faced reality quite resolutely at all times and retains a wry sense of humour despite extreme circumstances. I have seen no evidence of depression throughout my contact with her. She is sad about her illness and situation but this does not equate to clinical depression.

After two prolonged consultations, it was clear to me that Susan's quality of life was being severely damaged by the toxic anxiety associated with her uncertain prognosis, and her fear regarding her future. I had no hesitation in providing her with two prescriptions for amylobarbitone, and advice about the drug, which would give her control over the end of her life. I also designed an advance directive for her.

As with others I have treated, I encouraged her to write down her thoughts. She responded in an eloquent and moving way.

The option of voluntary euthanasia is precisely that, an option. One I have considered fully and thoroughly. Though I regard my decision to obtain the means and assistance for me to take my own life as a way of regaining a sense of control, I realise that the desire to live is strong. It is a real possibility that I may be unable to take my own life because personal experience has led me to believe that as humans we can endure suffering that can seem unimaginable. I have endured more than I thought able and I think it is virtually impossible to determine when enough is enough. I have wondered what my limits might be, but I think it's entirely possible that I may reach those limits and reassess them. Nevertheless while there are questions as to the degree of suffering I am prepared to endure and whether I will be able to take my own life, it is important for me to be in a position whereby I can exercise my right to die in a manner determined by me. I don't want to be a mere shell of my former self. My greatest fear is that I will undergo drastic mental and physical changes so much so that I won't be me anymore. And what is even more distressing is that I may be trapped in a body that will not allow me to communicate with those I love and care for.

I believe that voluntary euthanasia offers me an opportunity to preserve me as a whole and complete person in the minds of others, which is very important to me.

Since obtaining the means by which I can take my own life at a time of my own choosing, I have felt an enormous sense of relief. There is a sense of relief not felt since [before] the time of my diagnosis of an inoperable brain tumour. In the eight years since being diagnosed, I have had to live with the fear and full knowledge of what may happen to me as a result of having a brain tumour. These thoughts have plagued me consistently over these last years and at times, many times, completely overwhelmed me.

I do feel a degree of anger that the last eight years have been plagued with unpleasant thoughts and anguish needlessly. My quality of life would have been far better had the medical establishment provided me with reassurance and respected my need to maintain some sense of control, when they themselves made it abundantly clear that the tumour would ultimately result in my death.

I continued to see and support Susan over the next two and a half years. Unfortunately, in late 2005, she developed rather rapidly progressive loss of feeling and power in her right leg, and her speech became slurred. Although she had the means to end her life, she battled on, accepting in-patient palliative care, where her advance directive ensured that her life was not prolonged by intrusive treatment, and she received sedation at the end.

I reflected on other comments in her letter to me:

Nevertheless while there are questions as to the degree of suffering I am prepared to endure and whether I will be able to take my own life, it is important to me to be in a position whereby I can exercise my right to die in a manner determined by me.

The fact that she did not take her own life is, to me, totally un-important. I had slowly begun to realise, and this experience clarified it, that at no point was it my intention that Susan should end her own life. In most circumstances where I had provided advice and medication, the intensity of the suffering and the immediacy of the situation had led to rapid action, leading me to think that I was assist-ing their suicide. But Susan's two-year delay and eventual death within palliative care put this very clearly in another perspective. My intention had been to make the option of a self-administered death possible, if she chose it, and by making it possible to enhance her quality of life. I think her letters make it clear that having the option available to her did enhance the quality of her life. I suspect that her relatively young age and her young children were important factors in her final decision.

In fact, what mattered to me was that she could make a choice, and that she chose a palliative care option was totally satisfactory to me. It is not the method by which people die that matters, but the manner in which they die—with what is, for them, dignity and without suffering. To do that they need choice. It is my ultimate aim to see physician-assisted dying become an integral part of palliative care, such that the very best of care will be available to all. I support pallia-tive care. No doubt the vast majority of people receiving palliative care are pleased with the outcome and do not seek assistance in dying. Most will find traditional palliative care totally adequate, but if they do not, they should be able to ask for something more. Only then will they have had available the very best choice of care, discussed in an open fashion, without strings attached and with their choice respected. Unfortunately, the present attitudes of some significant palliative care leaders make this unlikely.

In February 2007, Professor Margaret O'Connor, President of Palliative Care Australia (PCA), stated, 'I would have very few direct experiences of requests (for assisted dying) from people about it'.[1] She believed that debate about physician-assisted dying was premature until palliative care was available to all, despite PCA's position statement indicating that it could not provide complete relief of suffering!

Margaret O'Connor's statement is intriguing. Over the past ten years, I have received more than 500 requests for end-of-life assistance and advice. As an outspoken advocate for physician-assisted dying, and a counsellor for Dying With Dignity Victoria, I could expect to receive more than a minimal number of such requests. But why such a large discrepancy, when Professor O'Connor is herself so closely involved in palliative care?

Is her experience mirrored by other palliative care professionals? Breitbart and colleagues found that 16 per cent of chronically ill cancer patients receiving palliative care expressed a high level of desire for a hastened death.[2]

Does palliative care create a climate that is intimidating to such requests? Is there some selection process whereby certain individuals deliberately avoid engagement with palliative care through fear of diminished control?

I do not know the answers to these questions, but I do know two facts. First, that palliative care is uncomfortable with such requests and tries to deflect them, and second, that it says it is not able to relieve all the pain and suffering of its clients. And yet that would not be entirely true if palliative care were to employ terminal sedation in a more liberal and significantly aggressive fashion. Palliative care seems reluctant to talk about terminal sedation, some experts even denying the necessity for its use, and others using it with great reluctance. Others see terminal sedation as the palliative care answer to other forms of physician-assisted dying, but it is an inadequate answer.

Some readers may feel that I am antagonistic to palliative care. I am not. I am full of admiration of the tremendous work that they do. I support palliative care, but not completely. Most of their patients are fully satisfied with their help, but not all. It is palliative care's reluctance to fully acknowledge these patients and assist them of which

I am critical. Marcia Angell, former editor of the *New England Journal of Medicine*, summed this up, saying, 'I am also concerned that the hospice and palliative care movement, as it has grown in importance and influence, has developed a mindset typical of many specialized disciplines, a professional pride that borders on hubris and rigidity'.[3]

Angell went further, saying that the palliative care ideal (model) of the good death

> does not leave much room for patients for whom control and independence are highly important. I have even heard such people disparaged as overly controlling—as though they should somehow get with the program and die right. But it is wrong to assume that all people will approach death in the same way. Some will, indeed, become ideal hospice patients, but others will rail against the dying process until the end, and they will want that end to come sooner. They too are human. We should be careful not to impose our views of a good death on others.[4]

I quote the palliative care literature widely to demonstrate how difficult it is to provide complete relief of all pain and suffering. I am not surprised at this. I do not emphasise this to damage palliative care, but to reveal the truth. I am also critical of terminal sedation in some contexts, because, in many situations, it is the doctor's solution to the problem, but not one that their patient would choose if they had an option. As Professor Michael Ashby says, 'Palliative care is a model of care, not a moral crusade, and should not be used as a strategic weapon in social debates'.[5] Such a model of care cannot possibly be acceptable to everyone, nor should everyone be forced to accept such a model because of palliative care's refusal to embrace an alternative.

In some ways, a dying person could be seen as someone trapped in their room on the sixteenth floor of a hotel that is on fire. Palliative care is the fire brigade that is endeavouring to put out the fire and rescue the dying person from their suffering. Most hotels have a fire escape, which in the last resort allows relief from the terror. In the palliative care hotel the fire escape is locked, which means that if the fire brigade cannot put out the fire, there is no escape. Physician-assisted dying is the key to the fire escape when palliative care fails.

19

STEVE GUEST

A Death Not in Vain

'I have learned from my life in medicine that death is not always the enemy. Often it is good medical treatment. Often it achieves what medicine cannot achieve—it stops suffering.'
Dr Christiaan Barnard, *Good Life, Good Death*

On Monday morning, 11 July 2005, I left the Voluntary Euthanasia Society of Victoria office shortly after 10 a.m. My car radio is permanently tuned to 774 ABC (Melbourne), and I caught the tail end of Jon Faine's talk-back segment. I was excited because the calls were about the right to die with dignity. I wondered what had set this off.

That same evening I found out. I had a phone call from Steve Guest,[1] a 58-year-old man seeking my help. I did not know him nor had I spoken to him before this. He was the person who that morning had rung Jon Faine, the program's erudite presenter, and generated the discussion. He had rung to say that he had incurable cancer and to express his anger at those religious people who prevented him receiving the same compassionate help to die as his canine companion had, and to advocate for a change to the law.

Some seven weeks before this, his brother, John Guest, had written to the journalist Terry Lane, who regularly appears on Faine's program. John had written as follows.

> You might like to speak to a man I know well. He's 58, intelligent, articulate, and dying of an inoperable cancer which might give him two or three months to live, perhaps a bit more. He hasn't eaten for six months and feeds himself gunk through a tube arrangement implanted in his stomach. He's gone from 85 to 50 kg but his mind is clear and his sense of humour undiminished. He sees his illness as a statistical abnormality, luck of the draw.
>
> He wants his death to be in a time, place and manner of his choosing, which means at home with his books and a couple of friends when he gets to the point where the pain is too much and/or he has to be placed in a hospice. He has been to one of Philip Nitschke's seminars but was told effectively: Sorry, but all I can tell you is that I mustn't tell you anything. This means he'll have to take his own steps with whatever help he can get from sympathetic parties.
>
> He'd like to talk to someone such as yourself about one particular aspect of his position. He regards his life as his own and is resentful of the religious rump that believes it's theirs. He believes he has every right to leave it and objects to their requirements that if he insists on going he must do so gruesomely (to borrow from your piece today). He carries no religious baggage himself and accepts that death is a better alternative than a prolonged and continuously worsening life of pain, misery and indignity. But they won't let him if they can stop him.

It is quite clear from this letter that Steve Guest had made up his own mind to end his suffering at some point—he needed no incitement from anyone.

Terry Lane did contact Steve, and his brother believes they spoke at length on two occasions in July. He also believes that Lane suggested Steve call me. Lane may have suggested that he ring Jon Faine's talk-back program. In any event, Steve did ring Jon Faine, and immediately grabbed his attention. The usual talk-back call lasts only one to two minutes, but Steve's call engaged the next ten minutes, and the talk-back air-waves then became swamped by sympathetic responses and tragic end-of-life stories. It was as though a dam wall had broken. It was riveting, spontaneous radio. Steve's message was that he had no control over his death, and he believed that government, in thrall to the religious hierarchy, denied him that control.

I was blissfully unaware of all this when I returned Steve's phone call, but the penny dropped after a few moments. After I had talked to Steve for about forty-five minutes, I had a clear picture of a man in great distress, who deserved to be treated with respect and compassion. In my opinion he needed urgent care. He was immobile due to his illness, so I agreed to drive to his home at Point Lonsdale, some 90 km away, and meet him the next morning.

I did not park any distance away from his home, as I had done in 1993 with Alice (chapter 6) out of fear of discovery. My experience over the past twelve years had minimised that fear, and in the back of my mind was an idea that this might be a situation over which a challenge to the status quo might be mounted. Perhaps Steve and I had been destined to meet.

I found Steve to be haggard and drawn, in keeping with a man who had lost a great deal of weight in a few months, and who was suffering from terminal cancer. His story began nine months before when he had noticed difficulty in swallowing. Investigation revealed a blockage to his gullet (oesophagus) by cancer. An operation confirmed this, but also revealed that the cancer could not be removed due to invasion of surrounding structures, including the body's main artery, the aorta. Without any prior discussion (but not unreasonably), a stomach tube (PEG) was placed for future feeding. A course of radiotherapy and chemotherapy, predictably, had no effect on the progress of this most unresponsive tumour.

Now, nine months on from that operation, Steve existed by virtue of the artificial liquid 'food' supplement that he injected into his stomach via his PEG. Despite this, he had lost more than 35 kg. His cancer had taken over his metabolism and he was declining rapidly. He was aware that he was approaching death and that he had only weeks to live. He had an extremely good relationship with his local doctor, and was receiving excellent care. His family was aware of his situation and was very supportive. As he grew weaker, this network of family and friends was becoming more important.

As I talked to Steve over a two-hour period, I became aware of a complex web of physical, psychological and existential issues that were causing him intolerable and, it seemed, unrelievable suffering. Steve had physical pain in his upper right back, or shoulder blade area, which was due to infiltration of the cancer into the chest wall in this area. In order to control this pain, he was using a morphine patch with liquid morphine for breakthrough pain. He had to instil this liquid morphine through his stomach tube. Whilst the morphine gave him reasonable although not complete relief from this pain, that relief came at considerable cost. The morphine caused distressing nausea and severe constipation requiring enemas for bowel comfort. The worst side-effect of the morphine was severe mental clouding, when he wished to be alert and creative. He said that 'it felt like he had an injection of lead into his brain'. Going hand in hand with his weight loss was a profound lack of physical energy—extreme weakness—such that it was difficult to stand, and walking more than a few yards caused major exhaustion. He had no appetite, which was perhaps just as well, as he had no ability to swallow and therefore enjoy the taste of food and drink.

This leads into the psychological distress. Even the simple pleasures of life that most take for granted were denied him. Eating, drinking, the pleasures of tasting food and exercising were impossible.

His ability to concentrate was impaired, making thinking, conversation and reading difficult. But far more important were more abstract psychological issues. As he said to Jon Faine, 'My days are awful'. He was facing a complete loss of control over the circumstances of his life. He was just managing to maintain himself in his own home with the help of his brothers, his friends and the community. But very soon this would no longer be possible, and he would face total dependence in hospital, hospice or a nursing home. This was a complete anathema to him. These psychological issues crossed over the border into existential distress, a distress related to the threat to those things that made Steve who he was. His very existence as a human being was being destroyed, but while he remained alive. His sense of dignity, his sense of worth and his reason for being was at threat. Steve was a proud, independent man and to die in circumstances where he simply faded away slowly, being ministered to for every need by people he did not know, no matter how kind, was not, to him, dignified. His certain mode of death was by cachexia, a starvation caused by the cancer, a slow wasting death, each meaningless day followed by another even more dependent. In addition there was likely to be a crescendo of pain and other physical symptoms at the end—'when dying patients experience a crescendo of unmanageable suffering in the last days of life'.[2]

Such a mode of dying cannot be palliated. His pain could be only partially eased, but at significant cost. His need for morphine would inevitably escalate as his pain increased and he developed tolerance to the drug. It would get worse, and so would the side-effects. His wasting was unalterable by any palliation.[3] The best palliative care could offer for his psychological distress was 'supportive counselling and [consideration] of benzodiazepines'.[4] He was not receptive to the former alone, and the latter would simply increase his intellectual disintegration. In my opinion his psychological suffering could not be altered by traditional palliative care, and his existential suffering was beyond salvage by the kind words of strangers. Reassurance that he would not be allowed to suffer cuts no ice in this situation. It requires specific information and medication if positive control is to be achieved, and the relief of suffering that goes with that. Formal palliative care had nothing to offer him. It was possible that if he fell into sympathetic palliative hands that he would be offered terminal sedation to ease his last hours or perhaps days, but he simply abhorred the idea of lingering on in a medically induced coma whilst in 'care'. I explained the possible benefits of palliative care, but he totally rejected the idea. He did not want his death to be medicalised by the continuous care that he would require. Steve was far from alone in considering ending his life in these circumstances. Nessa Coyle and her colleagues found that 'suicide' was openly discussed as an option by more than a quarter of advanced cancer patients with severe symptoms. Only a particularly severe degree of overall fatigue appeared to distinguish these patients from others.[5] This Steve had in spades.

Steve denied being depressed, and he clearly retained in his conversation a wry sense of humour. His GP did not see him as depressed. Despite his medication, his intellect and judgement were intact and his analysis of his situation was accurate. Jon Faine was so impressed by his 'coherence and lucidity' that he could not imagine that he was suffering! Jon had not at that stage met Steve in person. Steve had been married but had been separated from his wife for four years. He had twin 23-year-old daughters with whom he had shared his views and who fully understood and supported his desire to have control over the end of his life. His two brothers were fully informed and fully supportive. He had no lack of family and social support. He had an excellent GP who was attentive to his needs and sympathetic, but Steve had not felt it appropriate to discuss his end-of-life problem with him as it might have compromised him. Steve had no spiritual issues. He was an atheist, who had come through any anger and recrimination that he might have suffered to a state of acceptance, a state that is necessary to have any hope of a 'good death'. He now wanted the freedom to do things his way. He wanted control over the end of his life.

In my opinion, there was little I could do for his physical symptoms, but they were not his major problem. His major suffering was
his psychological and existential suffering due to lack of control over
the end of his life. That was something I could give him and, in my
opinion, that would be medical treatment of the utmost palliative
value. And the alteration of his psychological state would have a positive impact on his perception of his physical symptoms, particularly
his pain, because pain is ultimately appreciated in the mind, and the
psychological state is critical to the perception of pain.

Steve wanted to end his suffering on his own terms, at a time and
place of his choosing, and in a manner that he considered secure
and dignified. Steve did not want to die—in reality he did not want
to end his life—but he did want to end his suffering. I did not incite
him to do that, nor did I want to. What I wanted to do was to give
him maximal palliation and to respect his autonomy to make his own
decisions.

For Steve, going to the end of the road with the physical degra-
dation that may be involved, or being drugged to death slowly over a
number of days, would be completely lacking in dignity. Whilst many
people like Steve want to end their own lives, and are prepared to take
that responsibility, they do want security, certainty and dignity. Many
people try to end their lives by violent and gruesome means but are
not always successful. Even if they are successful, these methods totally
lack dignity and leave a huge residue of grief for their loves ones. For
security and dignity one needs medical advice and prescription. Dignity
in dying is of fundamental importance to virtually everyone, and may
be hard to find in many deaths. Moreover, dignity is a very personal
concept, differing quite widely in the minds of different individuals.

Steve's concept of dignity was something personal, special to him,
internal. What he considered to be dignified might be different to my
perception, but for him, it was 'indivisible from his core being and
essence'.[6] He did not hold with a remote universal concept that
everyone has inherent dignity that persists no matter what their

circumstances. This universal concept, sustained by some idea of natural law, is much loved by religion and advanced to oppose the hastening of death, but Steve had no truck with religion.

Steve felt acutely that he was losing his dignity, but realised that he could retain it in two ways: first, by making a proud, purposeful, personal public statement during his remaining time and, second, by taking responsibility and control over the end of his life.

Steve and I discussed all this in great detail, and at the end he had persuaded me that his need for control was not only the most important medical need that he had, but it was also the most important thing I could do for him as a human being. I therefore answered all his questions and provided him with advice and medication that would allow him to end his life, should he choose, with security and dignity.

Because of distance it was difficult for me to visit Steve, but I phoned him five times over the next fourteen days to assess and support him. During this time, Steve undertook a media campaign that would have tired anyone, let alone someone with terminal cancer. He was energised by his new sense of control and his renewed sense of purpose. I visited him again on the morning of 26 July. He was so weak he could barely walk, and he was facing the imminent prospect of being unable to care for himself at home. He died that evening, in the company of his brothers.

For quite some time before I met Steve, I had formed the opinion that it might be a considerable time before Victorian politicians had the moral courage to address the issue of choice in dying with dignity. They were more concerned about retaining or gaining office to risk adopting this issue for legislative reform, even if a majority of them personally believed that it was a proper thing to do. And there is no doubt that there are potential risks for a political party or politician that would support legislative change; however, there are also potential advantages. Nevertheless, I had formed the opinion that this issue was probably more likely to be resolved through the courts, as abortion had been way back in 1969. Then, Justice Menhennitt had ruled that an abortion was not criminal if it was performed to protect the life or health of the pregnant woman. To this day, the statute law in Victoria remains unchanged, essentially outlawing abortion, but Menhennitt's ruling established a precedent that effectively annulled the statute law. I was also reminded of the courageous behaviour of Dr Bertram Wainer and his colleagues, who had challenged the existing law on abortion.

My esteemed medical colleague and friend Professor Peter Baume, one-time minister in the Australian Federal Parliament, had also expressed the same opinion to me—that the law was more likely to change due to a legal precedent than from legislative reform. It was obvious that there was a reluctance to proceed with prosecution or apply penalty on lay persons accused of, or admitting to, 'mercy killing'. Baume felt that the same lack of penalty would continue for lay persons, but the question of a doctor aiding and abetting suicide had never been tested. This was the section of the *Crimes Act* (6B) that particularly inhibited doctors. My experience over thirty years with public statements and deliberate provocation had led me to believe that there was a reluctance on the part of police and prosecutors to pursue such matters. Would a medical test case change the course of practice in physician-assisted dying as it had changed the practice of abortion?

What would be necessary for a test case to have a chance of success? First, it would require an individual with important characteristics. It would require someone with a credible and compelling story of intolerable and unrelievable suffering due to a terminal illness. Further, that individual must have been able to clearly express the nature and extent of that suffering. That person must have intelligence, courage and determination to tell their story to the public, so that the issue would resonate in the community. They must be able to speak with integrity, to engage with the public and evoke compassion. Above all, that individual must be able to convince the public of their rationality, of their coherence and of the clarity of their decision; that it was their decision, uninfluenced by others, and that they totally owned it. In this respect, a public profile and a visual and aural record of his circumstances before that person died would be invaluable. Second, it must be clear that the individual had benefited from the advice that they were given, that it had enhanced the quality, and perhaps the quantity, of their life, and had a palliative value. Third, it would be necessary to develop a sound legal argument that the advice was not incitement, that it was given to a rational person with the intention of palliation, and that the person derived benefit. For years it had been assumed that providing someone with the means to end his or her life would be unequivocally seen as aiding and abetting suicide, that the glass was unarguably full. Over the years that I had been advising people, I had come to see this glass as only 'half full', and consequently as 'half empty'—that one could view the same circumstances as 'half full' (aiding and abetting) or 'half empty' (providing good palliation). Finally, it would require a doctor to report the giving of advice in order to provoke the challenge.

As I drove for ninety minutes to see Steve, I was pondering if Steve was the right person, but also whether I had the 'balls' to risk the challenge. I was well aware of the possible effect on my ability to practice medicine, but I was in the twilight of my career. I realised that it would have significant effects on my family, on my social milieu and on possible financial consequences. But the greatest consequence would be on my emotional and physical state. Daryl Stephens, the Perth urologist who was charged with the murder of his patient, was a personal friend of mine, and I was aware of the stress he had to endure.

After speaking to Steve for more than two hours, I was convinced that he was the right individual around whom a challenge could be based. He had all the necessary characteristics—he had clearly indicated that he wanted to end his suffering before I met him. He had gross suffering that was readily apparent. He was intelligent and courageous. He was media savvy and had already demonstrated his desire to make his mark publicly.

Thus, only after I had both pledged my support and given him the advice he wanted did I explain how valuable his commitment could be. I did not want his participation to be contingent upon my decision to treat him. There was a further aspect. I strongly believed that if he had a target for achievement over the last days or weeks of his life, then his sense of purpose would be greatly enhanced and his quality of life significantly improved. Steve had already spoken to Jon Faine about a further program, and he was very ready to talk to any journalist who was interested. Philip Nitschke was arranging for him to speak at an EXIT meeting in nearby Geelong. I had been involved in the filming of a documentary about attitudes of dying people, and Steve agreed to talk to the film-maker. Kate Legge, the excellent journalist with *The Australian* who specialises in social and aged care issues, visited Steve and published an excellent piece. A local journalist with the *Geelong Advertiser*, Rebecca Tucker, became involved. Jon Faine's second interview with Steve ran for an hour and was arresting radio. The listening public was completely engaged.

With all this media exposure, there was now a large body of evidence as to Steve's state of health and of mind, and of the effect of my advice upon his condition. I felt confident enough to ring Kate Legge and tell her that I had 'given Steve advice that gave him control over the end of his life'. I repeated this comment subsequently to Rebecca Tucker and to Lorna Edwards of *The Age*, and rang Jon Faine's talk-back segment to make the same comment. I wanted it to be widely known that I had visited Steve and given him advice, but without being specific about that advice. That would dangle in the air, perhaps inviting the police to take an interest.

I first talked to Steve on 11 July. He died on 26 July. I met him on 12 July and spoke to him on five occasions during the next two weeks. I visited him on Monday 26 July in the morning for about two hours. He died that evening. I was not present, but his two brothers were. I was glad that they were there, first, and most importantly, to support him, but second, to provoke an answer to the mythical question as to whether loved ones who were present when a 'suicide' occurred were considered to be guilty of aiding and abetting that event (the Nancy Crick question). Steve's death was referred to the coroner, not unexpectedly in view of all the media comment, and the autopsy, I believe, revealed the presence of barbiturates in his blood.

There was relative calm for the next six months, until in early January 2006 I had a call from two gentlemen from the Victorian Homicide Squad informing me that they wished to interview me in relation to Steve Guest's death. On my questioning, they stated it was a suicide due to an overdose of barbiturates. My heart raced and missed a beat or two when I opened the door to these men. I was not sure whether it was from fear or the excitement of realising that the challenge had begun. The interview was to be a formal occasion at a later date in the Crime Squad headquarters, and they informed me that a videotape of the interview would be made available. It struck me that this was a very good opportunity to record my side of the story, whilst retaining the right to refuse any questions that did not appeal to me. I prepared a careful statement and read that onto the record. The sergeant's questions were answered truthfully or ignored. The most humiliating aspect of the visit was having my fingerprints taken like a common criminal. I will admit to being common, but I am no criminal. Apart from this, the police were pleasant and courteous, even, I thought, a touch apologetic about the whole process.

Not long after this I watched the Australian climber Lincoln Hall interviewed by Andrew Denton on ABC television. This man had climbed to within a stone's throw of the summit of Mt Everest, but could go no further. He was as close to dying as one can go as a result of his endeavour, but he was determined to go back and reach that summit, not because it was Mt Everest but because it was his 'Everest'. I somehow feel that Steve Guest is my 'Everest'.

In November 2006, the documentary *Do Not Resuscitate* was shown on SBS television. This provided an excellent aural and visual record of

Steve, his views, his illness and its devastating effects, of my relationship with Steve, and of the effects on him of having control. In it he spoke poignantly of his mental anguish, his corrosive anxiety and his fear regarding the manner of his death.

By March 2007, there had been no further action. The police had last spoken to Steve's brother John seven months earlier. I arranged an interview with Lindy Burns (ABC radio) and indicated that I had given Steve advice about barbiturates, about dose, about their effects and how to use them. In April, I was invited to appear on the SBS TV documentary program *Insight* on *Dying with Dignity*, and repeated those exact statements. It was now clearer what 'giving Steve control over the end of his life' entailed.

On 22 June 2006, Dying With Dignity Victoria held a public rally on the steps of Parliament House to remember Steve Guest as a symbol of courage and of the right to die with dignity. I spoke to that rally about my relationship with Steve, repeated my comments about barbiturates and added that I had given him medication. My involvement with Steve's death was spelt out in my article that morning in the opinion page of *The Age* newspaper. When the police were invited to comment, they stated that the investigation was continuing. Six months later, nothing more had been heard from them. It was now nearly two and a half years since Steve's death and the coroner had yet to hold an inquest. Steve's brother John had been informed by the police that the inquest would probably be 'closed'—that is, not calling witnesses and not open to the media. I seem to remember phrases such as 'justice delayed is justice denied', and 'justice seen to be done'.

The police brief of evidence, prepared at the request of the coroner, was finally handed to the coroner late in 2007. The coroner then asked the Director of Public Prosecutions for an urgent opinion on the brief. Shortly after, in January 2008, the coroner wrote to Steve Guest's brothers explaining that an inquest would not be held until after any criminal charges had been dealt with. The coroner is now asking the police whether they are intending to lay any charges. No one, it seems, is very keen to deal with this matter.

In the meantime, I had seen another person with bulbar type MND (early effect on swallowing, speech and breathing). I had no hesitation in providing Peter with advice and medication, and he and his wife were keen to speak out about their dilemma. In October 2007, I had the opportunity to talk in depth to journalist Julie Anne Davies of *The Bulletin* magazine.[7] A flagrant cover resulted, with the banner head-line 'Arrest me' plastered across my smiling photo with outstretched pleading hands! This left no doubt as to my intention to challenge the current status of the law. My journey had now almost run its course.

The question that I return to as I near the end of this book is this— is voluntary euthanasia a crime? When I first acted to relieve intolerable suffering, I was very concerned that it was so. Four decades later, I fancy it is not.

As a trivial matter, euthanasia is not mentioned in the statute law in Victoria that deals with assistance in suicide or intentional hastening of death (the *Crimes Act 1958*). Interestingly, the word is not mentioned in the recent legislation in the Netherlands that decriminalises these matters. That law simply makes legal the 'termination of life on request' under prescribed circumstances. Since the word 'euthanasia' has no accepted definition, it is not a good basis for legal process. So in this sense, 'euthanasia' is not illegal. It is a crime by statute in Victoria to cause death by intention (murder) or with foresight (manslaughter), and it is a crime to incite another person to commit suicide (the words in the *Crimes Act*) or to aid or abet another person in the commission of suicide. However, in the application of this law, it is recognised that doctors face unusual and difficult circumstances that create a vari-ation in legal practice. In 1957 in an English court, Justice Devlin, in *R v. Adams*, instructed the jury that 'the giving of drugs to an elderly patient to alleviate pain was lawful even if incidentally it shortened the patient's life'.[8] This is an application of 'double effect' reasoning in a legal rather than a moral sense to foreseeing the likelihood or con-sequence of medical treatment in hastening death. It allows many medical acts to be tolerated, whereas in non-medical circumstances the same foreseeing of a fatal consequence is not tolerated.

Thus, the defence in many medical acts that terminate life by an injection, or series of injections, is that the intent is to palliate. Why should the same defence in principle not also apply to the prescrip-tion of oral, rather than injectable, drugs?

One of the most destructive features associated with dying is the potential for cruel and debilitating anxiety associated with the psy-chological and existential suffering. It accompanies most people to some extent in this phase of their life. It is best summed up as a loss of control over their life at a very important time. The stories related in this book reveal this repeatedly. People are usually asked to trust complete strangers (the palliative care team) who they may sense have a fundamentally different, perhaps antagonistic, view of life from their own. For example, Ellen McGee writes, 'Hospice maintains that it has a vision of good dying; it presents an ideal of continued care, of valu-ing the individual even when he does not value himself'.[9]

Whenever we lack control over our lives, we suffer anxiety until that control is restored. How much more important is control when we are approaching the final moment of our lives, when how we die and where we die is fundamental to finding closure? To be able to say goodbye to one's own family in one's own home is what most would want. It is not always possible when sudden events wash over us like a tsunami, but in many circumstances it is possible. It should be possible in most palliative care, but expert Dr Michael Barbato makes it quite clear that this is rare: 'He prepared for his death; he died in his own bed after saying goodbye to his wife and family. It was one of those deaths that we in palliative care hope to see but rarely do'.[10]

The control of this toxic anxiety is recognised by palliative care experts as important. Dr Nathan Cherny, who underwent training in palliative medicine in Melbourne, wrote:

This offer of sedation as a therapeutic option is often received as an emphatic acknowledgement of the degree of patient suffering. The enhanced patient trust in the commitment of the professional care-givers to their relief of suffering may, in itself, provide enough relief of patient and family distress to render sedation unnecessary.[11]

In other words, the relief of anxiety is of profound value in diminishing suffering at the end of life.

My own experience as shown in this book confirms this value. First, there is value in simply reassuring someone that they are talking to a doctor who respects their point of view. Second, there is even more relief in gaining a commitment to advice about end-of-life matters. That escalates when advice is actually given, but it is only fully achieved when the necessary medication is obtained or provided. The effects of this are quite dramatic. It is very effective palliation of a serious problem that cannot be often obtained in any other way.

Mrs Knight is a very good example of this. Initially, she was very relieved to have found someone with whom she could communicate, who respected her views and committed to support her. But she remained anxious until I gave her information about drugs and until she obtained them from her GP. However, she still was not calm until she had chapter and verse as to how she could use them to gain control over her own life. Nevertheless, she was able to carry on for eighteen months with this support. Margaret was exceedingly emotional when I first met her, but her demeanour changed completely on being reassured of support, and on being given knowledge. She battled on for eight months with this support.

The letters of Jim's daughter clearly describe his relaxed state after my visit and the provision of medication. Once again, the letters of Susan, and the comments of her family, confirm the profound relief at gaining control. Her remaining life, some three and a half years, was enhanced by that sense of control that she had gained. Victor was in despair when he presented with advanced MND. After obtaining advice and medication, he battled on for sixteen months, even consenting to a feeding tube, because he had control. Steve Guest, although he only lived two weeks after he gained control, was profound testimony of the value of having control. He was able to fulfil his destiny in a most profound way as a result. There was a real possibility that one or more of these people would have taken violent action to end their life sooner if they had not been in control. While the provision of advice is important, many people will not feel really secure until they have medication that they can rely upon. Keith is an example of this. While I reassured him of my support, I did not give him specific advice and medication that he could rely on, and he subsequently took his own life without my aid. His distress was not relieved by what he may have thought to be platitudes. The provision of medication and advice has, in my opinion, a profound palliative effect for many people.

Numerous surveys have been conducted of the practices of Australian doctors in end-of-life situations, and all reveal that assisted dying by intentional drug overdose, 'assisted suicide' or lethal injection are common and persistent practices.[12] Roger Magnussen's book, *Angels of Death*,[13] reveals a common practice of assisted death within the HIV/AIDS community. Yet during this 30-year period, there has been only one prosecution of a doctor for assisted dying (Dr Daryl Stephens in West Australia), and this only after the Director of Public Prosecutions overrode the decision of a lower court magistrate not to prosecute. One could be forgiven for thinking that there is an unacknowledged benign 'conspiracy' to avoid prosecuting doctors for actions taken to relieve suffering at the end of life, and that no action will be taken unless it simply cannot be avoided by virtue of a complaint by a party closely related to the event. The conspiracy involves the knowledge that such events take place, and the understanding that it is necessary that they take place for the proper relief of intolerable suffering. Melbourne University Professor of Law Loane Skene put it this way: 'The difficulties in securing convictions are quite apart from the general disinclination of prosecutors to take action against doctors "doing their best" in an area where the law is often unclear (*and, perhaps, deliberately kept unclear*)[14] (my italics). Law Lecturer Margaret Otlowski confirmed that 'It is evident from this analysis of mercy killing cases that a glaring gap exists between the law in theory and the administration of the law in practice'.[15]

Those involved understand that the law is being manipulated to maintain a status quo that allows doctors to help their patients to die without being prosecuted. Otlowski again: 'The second matter for concern is that the enormous discrepancy between the law in theory and the law in practice threatens to undermine public confidence in the law and bring it into disrepute'.[16]

What is in operation is a 'Clayton's law', a law that appears to be a law, but does not operate as such. It is actually an abuse of the rule of law, but it works in an imperfect way, and it is believed that to change the law to regulate such practice would be too politically divisive and would rouse powerful religious forces. Our politicians do not seem to have the stomach for such a fight, just as they did not over the issue of abortion in the 1960s. In that instance, their bacon was saved by the ruling of Mr Justice Menhennitt in Victoria, which has allowed abortion to be practised openly and with care in Victoria for more than thirty years whilst it remains a crime in the statute book.

However, because of the absence of a 'Menhennitt' ruling about assisted dying, when such assistance is provided, it is almost always provided covertly. Therefore, the assistance, being deliberately concealed from scrutiny, may not be occurring with due care. Roger Magnussen describes a number of 'botched' attempts in his book, and of 'assistance' rendered by a wide range of people—from a variety of doctors (palliative care specialists, oncologists, other specialists, general practitioners), nurses, psychologists, counsellors and even a funeral director! Some were experienced, and some were very naïve. The range of drugs and methods used was extensive and largely seemed to depend on what was at hand. Second opinions and psychiatric opinions were non-existent—the only 'saving grace' was that most of the events seemed to be voluntary. My own early naïve attempts indicated to me that without guidance (through experience, research and particularly training) poor practice can occur in the use of drugs both in type and in quantity, let alone indication. And the 'conspiracy' creates sufficient fear in the minds of sympathetic practitioners to deter prescription of the most appropriate medications, and to encourage 'cocktails' of easily available drugs that may be insufficient, inadequate or downright harmful. In this respect, the situation bears some resemblance to that which existed in 'backyard' abortion before Menhennitt. My own experience is littered with requests from desperate people who have already made an inadequate and disastrous attempt to commit suicide on their own using stored medications without appropriate advice, and who, as a result of that horror and failure, were seeking effective guidance. It was not always possible to give it.

20

DYING WITH DIGNITY

*'Must one also pay for righteous acts? Was there another measure
besides that of reason?'*
Arthur Koestler, *Darkness at Noon*, 1940

*'The current two-tier system—a chosen death and an end to pain
outside the law for those with connections, and strong refusals for most
other people—is one of the greatest scandals of contemporary practice.'*
Professor Ronald Dworkin et al., The Philosophers' Brief, 1997; to
the US Supreme Court

*'As the law stands, only the good sense of prosecuting authorities and
juries stands between compassionate and courageous medical
practitioners and convictions for murder.'*
Richard McGarvie (State Counsel, Victoria)

I n this book, I have described a number of medical encounters
extending over a 35-year period. There are some common threads
that run through most of them. All of them involve people with

terminal illness or hopeless illness and who had intolerable and unrelievable suffering—intolerable as far as they were concerned, and unrelievable except by their deaths. The desire for a hastened death, in order to relieve their suffering, was explicitly expressed at the time by all except two. One clearly expressed his wish through his appointed agent, another through a legally appointed guardian. I was involved in hastening the death, in various ways, of all except four. This was achieved by giving advice and support to some and, to this extent, assisting them to end their own lives; for others by also providing medication that allowed them to end their own lives. In other circumstances assistance was by providing aggressive medication by terminal sedation for relief of symptoms, clearly foreseeing that death was a likely, and secondarily welcomed, outcome. A variety of means was used (but never a direct lethal injection) with a common outcome, reached through dialogue with the suffering person, or (if not possible) their appointed agent. The outcome was a relief of suffering; at a minimum 'the least worst death', but hopefully a 'good death'—that being the sufferer's intention. In essence, this was voluntary euthanasia according to my definition, that may be achieved in a variety of ways, and not, as many so-called authorities see it, only by a direct lethal injection.

A journey of discovery and learning

This book therefore describes a journey of discovery and learning, a journey that goes into the deeply personal feelings of people facing death, and a journey that discovers how such people may be helped, if one can be convinced of their real need for that help and is prepared to take small risks on their behalf. It was a journey stimulated by the suffering of severe pain and severe breathlessness, and progressing on to a wider view of suffering in the psychological and existential areas.

Recently, when browsing in the *British Medical Journal*, I read this comment by assistant editor Tessa Richards:

Are we [doctors] equally well prepared for dying and death? Speaking for myself, the answer is no. I dodged the issue before my own life-threatening surgery, and floundered as I witnessed my father's slow decline from dementia. Practising medicine conferred familiarity, but not understanding, competence or even compassion. I learnt a lot through following his journey. Not from the half-dozen doctors he was nominally under, but from his nursing auxiliaries, who without exception came from poor countries.[1]

She could have been describing me before I commenced this journey. I too have learnt from nurses, but more by listening to my patients. Sadly, medical education does not adequately prepare the young doctor for his or her journey, and some do not learn, or do so slowly, from the experiences that they meet.

It has been a journey in which I believe I have undergone a metamorphosis, in which I have retained the body of a urological surgeon, but have grown new wings—those of an (eccentric) palliative care physician and a psychological counsellor. I believe that this journey enables me to say something relevant about voluntary euthanasia. I have read copiously about the subject, listened to and debated with many. However, I find that many who write and talk about this subject have not had this journey; they have not even taken the first step of discussion of the possibility. Their first step is of denial. They talk from theory, from an ivory tower, about what they think voluntary euthanasia is about, but not what it actually is, or what it could be if legalised. Professor Margaret O'Connor, President of Palliative Care Australia, and one of Australia's leading authorities on palliative care research, has a profound opposition to physician-assisted dying. Despite having presumably nursed many thousands of dying patients, she said, 'Certainly, I would have very few direct experiences of requests from people about it'.[2] An expert with virtually no experience in such requests. A recent paper considered such requests as 'merely a passing comment that is not intended to be literally heard as a death wish'.[3]

Like Linda Emanuel, these are experts in denying the reality of such requests, and in deflecting them.[4] These are 'experts' in the subject but with no practical experience, akin to an academic Professor of Surgery who has never operated upon anyone.

A period of naivety and struggle

This history starts in 1974, with a seminal and thought-provoking moment with Betty. She stimulated my conscience, through emotions of guilt and shame, anger and frustration, to a belief that, as a doctor, I had a duty to respect autonomy and to relieve suffering, if requested. This was first expressed through aggressive relief of respiratory distress for a family member. In 1976, my hasty, naïve and ill-considered assistance to Len, and his undignified death, brought me abruptly to face two consequences. First, that it required a much more considered approach to these matters in order to help people with security and dignity, and, second, that providing such help was potentially a crime of serious proportions. Thus my conscience was pushing my behaviour in a direction that seemed to involve a crime by legal definition.

Fortunately, patients like Betty and Len are not common in a urological practice, but over the next sixteen years I treated other patients with incurable cancer, with lethal obstruction of the kidneys, to whom I gave advice regarding non-intervention, and traditional palliation was given. I had no requests in this time for assistance in dying, sparing a conflict between conscience and crime. The matter of euthanasia was often in my thoughts as the subject erupted in the media periodically, largely through events in the Netherlands. There the debate was predominantly about voluntary euthanasia by lethal injection rather than by 'physician-assisted suicide'; whereas my own thinking, based entirely on my clinical experience, led me very strongly to a preference for physician-assisted dying by self-administration.

I first entered the debate about voluntary euthanasia in 1987, believing that law reform was necessary in Australia.[5] My public revelation in 1992, and again in 1995, that I had assisted people to die led to a dramatic change in my situation. Whereas previously I had been infrequently exposed to the necessity to consider physician-assisted dying for my own patients, I was now receiving requests from strangers with non-urological conditions.

Should this make a difference? If a drowning man calls for help, should you help him if you know him, but not if he is a stranger? I think you should help, and these people were found to be drowning and bereft of help from those people who were supposed to be treating them.

Alice, Mrs Knight and Margaret were examples of this. Alice fully tested my conscience and resolve, and posed the problem of obtaining effective medication. Fortunately for Mrs Knight, her general practitioner prescribed the medication, but the questions she posed were those of timing and absence of depression. Margaret solved her own problem of method, and simply needed support and advice, but her death again drew attention to criminality. The lack of prosecution as an outcome actually suggested that the risk was not as great as it seemed.

Terminal sedation

From about 1990, I began to explore the medical literature on voluntary euthanasia, and came across the account of Diane by Timothy Quill. This led me to a union between my position derived from clinical experience and that of some bioethicists such as Helga Kuhse, Peter Singer, Margaret Pabst Battin and Ronald Dworkin, among others, who essentially reached a similar position from philosophical analysis. My chance discovery of the clinical use of terminal sedation in 1995 led me deeper into the palliative care literature, and a new picture of practice, 'not often discussed in an open fashion', emerged. This practice of terminal sedation seemed to have been rapidly and seamlessly absorbed into accepted palliative care practice and ethics, and to have gained quasi-legal status, surely because it filled a desperate need (relieving the otherwise unrelievable). As Dr David Asch said, 'Many clinicians who care for patients like this are probably gratified about the increasing acceptance of terminal sedation as a therapeutic approach in these situations'.[6]

At that time, I could see no essential difference between this practice and voluntary euthanasia except time and also, arguably, in some cases, consent and dignity. Others later dubbed it 'slow euthanasia', confirming my view.[7] Pamela, Jane and Howard were all people for whom 'physician-assisted suicide' was not possible, but who wanted assistance. Terminal sedation was a way of both helping them and bringing scrutiny to this process by way of the coroner. The reluctance of both the coroner and the Attorney-General to address the necessity to report such deaths strengthened my view that the authorities found this issue a difficult one, since accepted medical practice verged so close to 'criminal criteria'. Authorities were therefore reluctant to pursue any prosecution unless they were forced to do so by a highly specific complaint.

Through difficulty to reasonable practice

Interspersed with these instances of terminal sedation were difficult situations such as Keith and Helen. Not all voluntary euthanasia requests are straightforward, particularly without the benefit of second and expert opinions, as is, unfortunately, commonly the case in covert practice. Keith pre-empted my assistance—I was too fearful, too slow, too cautious for him. We did not communicate well enough. He did not appreciate the difficulties involved in providing medication. I probably added to his suffering by my delay. But there is a need for caution, for a feeling of surety, even certainty, and even more so in a slowly progressive, hopeless illness compared to a terminal illness. Jane waited seven months whilst I became certain and found a way. Helen waited three months to convince me that her blindness and threatened incarceration in a nursing home were sufficient suffering to justify assisting her in a more direct way. Her family doctor prescribed for her, but I helped her prepare her 'cocktail', since, being blind, she could not do this with security. With most assisted suicides, the physician's involvement is with counselling, advice and prescription, but in this covert era, the doctor is not usually present when death occurs. I was impressed by the calm certainty of this mature and courageous woman as she prepared to end her life. Some, not knowing her, might think her reasons, and her suffering, insufficient. Suffering is personal and contextual, and it is condescending to doubt another's suffering without decent inquiry. She, and I, had no doubt.

Jim and Victor represented what for me was effective medical assistance in dying: clearly defined disease with undoubted intolerable and unrelievable suffering, effectively ended by the individual with security and dignity, the only sadness being that the whole matter was covert and that some had to die alone. Frank was beyond my skills and experience, while Susan accepted palliative care having been sustained by the provision of control. Michael's story saw the proper use of the *Medical Treatment Act* with refusal of treatment and maximal relief of pain and suffering. The journey had almost run its course. It moved closer with Steve Guest.

Patient profiles

Of the fifteen people assisted, six suffered from terminal cancer, five from progressive and ultimately fatal paralysis, one from a severe and usually fatal stroke, one each from heart and respiratory failure, and one was suffering from blindness in late life. Nine were suffering from terminal illness (within the difficulties of defining this term), whilst six had a hopeless illness. Surprisingly, there were no HIV/AIDS patients, yet these comprise a significant component of the requests in the Netherlands, where 22 per cent of these patients request voluntary euthanasia. This also supports the hypothesis of Dr Roger Magnussen that there is a network of medical and allied health care workers in Australia who are known to provide assistance to that community.[8]

The reasons for the request for assistance by this disparate group were wide and usually multiple. Pain was the major reason for the request in four, and a minor reason in six. Paralysis in various forms was a major factor in seven, but beyond the paralysis were loss of dependence, futility and loss of meaning and role. Other severe physical symptoms, including breathlessness and debility, were present in eight. Fear and anxiety, even terror, were significant emotional and psychological symptoms. However, most had significant existential suffering related to questions of dependence, burden, futility, loss of control, loss of meaning and role, and loss of dignity. To repeat what we have heard from Michael Ashby, Professor of Palliative Care at Monash University, when a person is suffering from the feeling of irretrievable loss of purpose and meaning from their life, it is not the role of the health-care team to suggest their care can reverse this.[9]

The stories in this book necessarily focus on suffering in the dying of a number of individuals. Because I have been involved with all of them in some way, it is inevitably also about me. However, my role is secondary. Their suffering and its relief are the core. Through the stories in this book, I have tried to illustrate the varying contexts in which medical assistance in dying can occur. At its simplest human level, it involves two people: a suffering person making a request and someone (usually, and in my view, properly, a doctor) responding with assistance. It has a simple personal context. It may also involve a varying number of close family, or friends, and there also may be a more distant medical and nursing circle of advisers and carers. In the vast majority of instances, no one beyond a handful of people at most will need to know just how a person actually died—it is a personal matter, not a community issue, whether someone dies naturally or by physician-assisted dying. Such dying does not require societal approval.

Once, while sitting on a sheer cliff at the most extreme tip of Cape Schanck watching albatross skimming the waves of Bass Strait, I contemplated the impact of my death if I fell from the cliff and drowned. My wife and children would be greatly affected and, to a lesser extent, my brothers; but while some people who know me would be saddened to hear such news, they would not be significantly affected, and within a few days I would fade from the daily memory of almost all people. Within a few days the ripples caused by my death would have stilled for all but a very few. The impact of a death is greatly altered by the age of the person and the circumstances. There is the world of difference between a young person succumbing in a violent and unexpected manner compared to an older person who has led a fulfilling life and whose death is expected. There is evidence that there is far less grief if that older person dies in a calm, controlled, peaceful and dignified manner, having accepted the reality of death.

Voluntary euthanasia with strict guidelines has now been practised in the Netherlands for twenty years. It has more than 90 per cent public support as an acceptable option. People in the Netherlands have proved to be far more worried that doctors might unduly prolong their lives with unnecessary treatment than that they might hasten their death without consent. There is not the slightest evidence that confidence in the medical profession has been harmed by allowing patients to request hastening of death and allowing doctors to respond under certain circumstances.

The stories in this book do not represent by any means the sum of people I have listened to, counselled, advised and assisted. They represent those for whom records and memory allow an accurate, and reasonably detailed, account. Some have been chosen because they have left eloquent and illustrative statements. The memory of most of these people will, for me, never dim. They have also been chosen in order to illustrate the wide context in which such dialogues take place, and the problems that exist in helping people in a theoretically hostile environment. Advice has been sought by people with a wide range of diseases and from many parts of Australia. Patients with cancer and severe neuropathic disease, particularly MND, have been the commonest, which is not surprising as it mirrors the Dutch experience. There, 10 per cent of cancer patients and 20 per cent of MND patients request voluntary euthanasia, compared to 2.7 per cent of people with other diseases.

Many requests have come from people suffering severe, chronic, unremitting pain from diseases affecting the skeleton, joints and muscles (the musculo-skeletal system). Chronic arthritis is a debilitating disease that is difficult to manage, and the constant pain is difficult to control. The side-effects of therapy can be severe in themselves. Eventually, such patients can simply become too tired to continue the fight to survive. Chronic spinal pain from injury or osteoporosis (thinning and softening of bone) is extremely difficult to treat and may be totally debilitating, preventing any normal activities and producing depression that can be resistant to therapy. Osteoporosis is a common accompaniment of the frailty of old age, and ultimately may threaten the ability of many elderly people, particularly women, to continue to live independent lives. They are desperately fearful of losing their independence and ending up in nursing home care, for them a fate worse than death.

Other prominent symptoms among people with serious requests have been those associated with very severe respiratory disease or heart failure, suffering from frightening breathlessness. They suffer from chronic anxiety, and panic, wondering where their next breath is going to come from, and knowing that there is no possible treatment available. Dr David Fishbein wrote, 'all too often … one is left with a patient with advanced cancer with severe dyspnoea, whose breathlessness is attributable to causes unresponsive to available treatment. The prospects for such patients are bleak and frequently dyspnoea persists until their demise'.[10] It is little wonder that Dr Martin Cohen stated that 'Dyspnoea however is probably an even more distressing symptom than severe pain'.[11] And what did Dr Fishbein advise in the way of palliation? 'Morphine in judicious doses should therefore be used in patients with widespread cancer and intractable dyspnoea not amenable to specific therapy to blunt the outgoing central motor demand.' For those not well versed in medical jargon, this means deliberately suppressing the ability to breathe with morphine, which relieves the symptom whilst 'killing' the patient (as happened with Ken in chapter 2).

But note, it must be judicious, for to do this too quickly in the course of events or too vigorously, even if that might better relieve the suffering, may result in raised eyebrows or accusations. So the effective relief of the patient's suffering may take second place to the interests of the doctor. It is no wonder that some people suffering from chronic breathlessness decide to take control of their own destiny rather then take their chance on finding that the doctor controlling their demise has no 'balls'.

There are many doctors who help patients like this to die in the security of their own home. I do not want to imply that I am alone in helping this group of patients. Some, however, whilst they believe in voluntary euthanasia in principle, do not want the law to change. They feel that they are practising good, humane and ethical medicine and do not want the law involved. But their attitude does not help those unfortunate people who are dying, with dyspnoea or other unrelievable symptoms, in public places where such assistance is less easily provided. More importantly, such activity should be open to public scrutiny and control, and they should be able to obtain second opinions and support from colleagues in making such important and often difficult decisions.

It is hard to think of a more compelling situation than a patient dying with severe breathlessness upon which to mount an argument for voluntary euthanasia. As Professor R G Twycross, the doyen of British palliative care, stated:

> Although firmly opposed to euthanasia, I consider that a doctor who has never been tempted to kill a patient probably has limited clinical experience or is not able to empathise with those who suffer … [and] a doctor who leaves a patient to suffer intolerably is morally more reprehensible than the doctor who performs euthanasia.[12]

It is extremely distressing and frightening for all involved—doctors, nurses, family and, most importantly, the patient. Conventional palliative medicine 'kills' such patients while saying that it is only intending to relieve the symptoms. Voluntary euthanasia practitioners say that they are relieving the symptoms and acknowledge that they are also 'killing' the patient. Professor Ashby gets around the point by this logic:

> It is sometimes argued that intentional shortening of life may be justified if requested by a terminally ill patient, and that so-called 'pharmacological oblivion' is merely a rationalisation of what the medical practitioner is really doing. However intentional ending of life is not part of palliative care practice and is different in kind from all other clinical intentions.[13]

In other words, it is all right to 'kill' me slowly but not abruptly. Such a semantic argument would be laughable except that it is central to the debate about physician-assisted dying. The patient is not laughing.

My philosophy towards end-of-life care

My philosophy towards end-of-life care has evolved over more than thirty years. It is based firmly on two interrelated principles—respect for the autonomy of a suffering person (their choice) and the necessity to relieve their suffering. Neither alone is totally sufficient, but when they combine they are compelling.

A person can express their autonomy only if they are fully informed about their clinical situation and about all the possible options for treatment or non-treatment. This can be a complex matter at the end of life and this is why I talk of the value of a dialogue between the person and their doctor to ensure that all issues are fully explored. Autonomy can be properly expressed only by a rational and fully informed person. Abnormal psychological or psychiatric factors must be sought and addressed, but my position is that a request for assistance is rational unless proved otherwise rather than the reverse. It is not for the patient to prove rationality any more than it is for the patient to prove competence (a similar issue) in such matters.

The issue at stake is the suffering of the patient, not the particular disease or its particular stage, whether it is terminal or not. For me, the patient must make the assessment of whether suffering is intolerable. I must assess whether anything can be done to relieve the suffering short of hastening death in terms of both physical and psychological domains. But it is not for me to judge the quality of life of the patient, or whether their life is worth living. That is entirely their decision. I firmly believe that a fully informed patient is in the best position to determine his or her best interests. This is not simply a medical matter as it involves the beliefs and values of the person, not those of the doctor. For the preservation of my own autonomy, I will need to be convinced that circumstances are present in which it is reasonable to expect intolerable suffering; alternately, that the suffering seems proportional to the stage of the disease and its present characteristics.

I do not accept the idea of voluntary euthanasia on demand, and therefore I must make a confirmatory judgement about the person's circumstances. If there is not synchrony between their position and mine, I will ask for time while assuring support. The person's request should never be snuffed out and the patient abandoned. Ultimately the patient owns the suffering, they own the right to request assistance, they own their fully informed and well-considered decision, they have the responsibility for the decision and own the consequences of that decision.

While I am committed to autonomy and the relief of suffering, it has always been my aim to support people on their life's journey as far as they can possibly go. There is no doubt that with support and care, people can often go further than they thought—palliative care shows that. A request for assistance is the start of a dialogue to determine the reasons for the request, to discover unmet needs and to assist only if there is no other reasonable option.

The essence of medical practice is the relief of pain and other suffering. Cure is of course a primary concern, but, at the end of life, care and relief of suffering is paramount. The failure to relieve pain and suffering at any time is improper, but at the end of life the relief of pain and suffering is the most important thing a doctor can do. There is a necessity to relieve that suffering, not a little, not gradually, but, in my opinion, to the extent and in the manner that is acceptable to the patient. Here is the link between the necessity to relieve suffering and the autonomy of the suffering person. If the maximal relief of suffering will threaten to, or will, hasten death, then the person must be informed of that. The person must be party to full and complete discussions as to the effects of maximal relief of suffering, as to the effects of a range of palliative treatments, and be able to choose between them. Whether it be a refusal of or withdrawal of treatment, the provision of death-hastening morphine, with or without coma-inducing sedatives, the provision of medication and advice to end life, or the delivery of a lethal injection, the choice should be with the individual. At the same time, the autonomy of the doctor must also be protected, and doctors cannot be expected to deliver a form of treatment that they find morally unacceptable. If there is intolerable and otherwise unrelievable suffering, relievable only by such an intervention, then the treatment is a matter of negotiation between the patient and the doctor. In my opinion, depending on the circumstances, any of the above treatment options may be considered to deliver a good death, so long as it is the choice of the patient, who considers that choice will bring a dignified death.

Readers will have noted that I have not described any instance where I have delivered what the Dutch would consider euthanasia; that is, a lethal injection by a combination of intravenous sedative and muscle relaxant. Nor have I ever done so. This is for four reasons. First, because I believe that, wherever possible, the responsibility for an end-of-life action should be with the person who decides to end their life. It is a great responsibility and I do not believe that it is proper to hand this to someone else when one can do it oneself. Second, euthanasia by lethal injection is seen as something done by someone (a doctor) to someone (a patient)—this diminishes the idea of control and responsibility of the person requesting the assistance. There is no more certain demonstration that the decision is voluntary and fully accepted than if it is completely owned, and acted upon, by the person with the suffering. The third reason is that there is no greater expression of personal autonomy than to control fully the timing and implementation (or not) of such a decision. Finally, I have never been confronted by a situation where the administration of a lethal injection was necessary. I believe that in the vast majority of situations where a valid request is made, that person will be capable of their own action. It is only if a person is totally paralysed, or unable to swallow or absorb oral medication, that an injection method would be necessary.

While I accept that advising and prescribing lethal medication to a person to enable them to end their life may be morally no different from providing a lethal injection, there is nevertheless a significant practical and emotional difference between these actions. Ultimately, there is far greater safety if the ultimate control over such action lies completely in the hands of the person desiring the action.

I am a doctor, not a bioethicist or philosopher. I approach these problems from a medical perspective, and regard such death-hastening acts on request as palliative acts. I see no medical distinction in providing maximal relief from intolerable suffering between terminal sedation, 'physician-assisted suicide' or a lethal injection. In the appropriate context, they are all palliative acts, the only distinctions being between time to death, the level of patient control and the intimate involvement of the doctor. Each action can provide what the person requests; each action can hasten death. They can all 'kill' a patient, if that is how one wants to see it. Terminal sedation, by creating some space between the onset of the action and the death, can provide what Jonathon Glover calls 'moral distance', which can be a comfort to some. For me, I find the deliberate use of terminal sedation, if it is prolonged, quite distressing, as may some patients and families. There is no doubt that, if that is the only option available, or the person specifically requests it, such action is gratefully accepted. I have no doubt, however, that if people had a real choice between terminal sedation on the one hand, and physician-assisted suicide or lethal injection on the other, that most would choose one of the latter. The distinction is between making a precise end with control and a clear mind, at home; and a slow, institutionalised demise in a blur of medication over an indefinite period of time. As to the choice between physician-assisted suicide and a lethal injection, I have not yet found anyone who did not accept that it was their responsibility to end their life, if that was their genuine wish and they were capable of doing so, with security.

This philosophy has evolved over thirty years. Its practice has provided me the most satisfying experiences of my medical career.

Consequences of the status quo

I have alluded to a 'conspiracy', which supports a status quo that allows assisted dying to go on in a completely arbitrary way, without scrutiny and without justice, and possibly without good reason or care. There is no doubt that some people can access assisted dying—a recent study of Victorian doctors showed that 35 per cent had 'administered medication, at the patient's request, with the intention of hastening death'[14] —but who are they, and how do they do it? First, they must be either lucky or well informed. They are lucky if their doctor has an understanding of the meaning of psychological and existential suffering. They are lucky if their doctor is affected by the experience of intolerable and unrelievable suffering and deliberately eases their death with large and frequent doses of analgesics, perhaps without any discussion; or lucky if their doctor is sensitive to their signals that they have had enough suffering and either wish to be eased or to commence a dialogue leading to assistance. They are lucky if their doctor is not morally affronted by hastening death in order to relieve otherwise unrelievable suffering, and is courageous enough to take some risk in bringing this about. They are lucky if they have had a prolonged relationship with a doctor who is open to discussion about end-of-life issues in a frank, non-judgemental way, and who believes in the ethical principles of autonomy and of the necessity to relieve suffering, and who commits in a non-paternalistic way to providing assistance at the end of life. They are lucky if they are dying in the privacy of their own home, where a sympathetic doctor can deliver drugs in safety, and sign the death certificate indicating that cancer or pneumonia was the cause of death. And they are lucky if another doctor, who countersigns the cremation certificate, sees no reason to 'stir the possum' if the death might have been a little premature or otherwise unexpected, but nevertheless inevitable. Moreover, they are lucky if they have a terminal disease that causes obvious pain that allows their doctor to prescribe large doses of analgesics, rather than a disease that causes severe psychological, emotional or existential suffering that is less well understood by most doctors, who are unused to terminal treatment with sedatives rather than analgesics. Luck plays a large part. They are unlucky if they are in the care of a doctor who is morally challenged by the slightest pos-sibility of hastening death and uses morphine in a cautious and restricted way, and regards terminal sedation as rarely necessary or, worse, as immoral.

If they are well informed, they will know that they can ask their doctor for aggressive relief of pain and suffering, and they will have family members who are prepared to be strong advocates for the ade-quate relief of their suffering. They will have discussed their wishes with their family and doctor, and have gained their understanding and support through their end-of-life journey. They will be able to make that time a worthwhile experience, secure in the knowledge that they have control over the circumstances of their dying in relation to when, where and how, to who will be present and to being able to say good-bye in a dignified manner. They will have been able to appoint an agent to protect their interests by refusing unwanted treatment if any event should render them incompetent, and will have completed an advance directive to make their wishes perfectly clear. They will understand their disease and their rights under the law, and know how to manage the medical situation to their advantage.

It clearly depends on who you are and whom and what you know. Doctors, dentists, veterinarians and pharmacists are privileged because of their knowledge and access to drugs, and all these groups have a much higher incidence of taking their own life than the general community. Dr Timothy Quill, who described the assisted death of Diana in 1991, recently wrote a retrospective titled 'Dying and decision making— evolution of end-of-life options', in which he described how he had helped his father to die. In it he said, 'Because our family understood how the system works and had knowledge and resources, we were able to use our fragmented health care system to provide him with comprehensive and humane end-of-life care. Most families are not so fortunate'.[15]

People with good education and positions of prestige and power have always been able to gain access to hard-to-obtain resources. I am sure that a Victorian premier or minister of health would be able to gain access to voluntary euthanasia, if they wanted it, more easily than the average citizen. Unfortunately, those of low educational and socio-economic status are far more likely to be ignorant of the law (such as the *Medical Treatment Act*), of voluntary euthanasia issues or to know how to gain access to, or argue, for assistance. Yet it is alleged that such groups will become the unnecessary victims of physician-assisted-dying legislation, because they will not be able to afford to seek good palliative care. That might be true in the deficient medical system of the USA, but in the universal health system in Australia it is not tenable. Another consequence of the status quo is the high incidence of often violent 'suicide' in older persons who cannot gain access to physician-assisted dying. The incidence of 'suicide' in older persons aged over sixty-five is twice that of the general population, and much of that is secondary to physical and existential suffering and the threat of loss of independence. It has never, however, been accurately quantified. What has been quantified is the toll of such unrelieved suffering and eventual 'suicide' on the widowers.[16] Investigators have quantified the 'caregiver burden' and the 'widower effect' on a survivor's health and find it to be very significant. However, the impact of a spouse's death on the survivor showed that giving a terminally ill spouse a 'good death'—one that is pain-free, one in which the dying person knows what to expect, and one in which they don't burden their loved ones—actually reduces the risk of death in the surviving partner.

A final consequence is the tragic 'mercy killings' that occur because no one will listen. Often, because of lack of sound information, the act fails, or if successful, the partner fails in a 'mercy killing pact'. The British Home Office has found that 30 per cent of mercy killers end up killing themselves in later life, haunted by the thought of their being driven to help a loved one.[17]

A criticism of my actions in this book could be that in many of these situations I did not have a significant patient–doctor relationship, and was not essentially the treating doctor—that I was in fact acting as a practitioner of medical euthanasia. I accept that criticism in part, but would argue that this was entirely due to the circumstances of covert practice. I totally accept that the appropriate place for physician-assisted dying is in the context of a solid patient–doctor relationship. However, this is not always possible, particularly when physician-assisted dying is viewed as illegal, and the suffering person cannot talk with their usual doctor. Even when legal, the primary doctor may have a moral objection to assisting that necessitates another doctor take on the responsibility. In my opinion, the ideal place for voluntary euthanasia is within the framework of palliative care, so that all the appropriate issues are addressed and all possible support given (without duress), but the patient is allowed to retain control of the process and to request assistance if the palliation provided is not adequate (not meeting their needs). This has been achieved in Belgium, where the impetus for legalisation of voluntary euthanasia has arisen from within an integrated palliative care system that realised that proper relief of suffering could not be provided by traditional palliative care alone. Further, in Oregon, physician-assisted dying by self-administration has been accepted by the hospice movement, and the majority of patients using this process are receiving hospice care.

In 2007, the American Academy of Hospice and Palliative Medicine took a neutral position on 'physician–assisted suicide'. One of its directors, Dr Nancy Hutton, said, 'I think it's taken as a way of providing comfort for unrelieved suffering. And so, in that respect, it would be consistent with a palliative care approach'.[18]

Unfortunately, there are some in Australian palliative care who see absolutely no circumstances in which voluntary euthanasia could be valid. These doctors and most other opponents of voluntary euthanasia hold their views on religious or moral grounds. They describe voluntary euthanasia as killing and therefore morally unacceptable. One could use the pejorative 'killing' for many medical acts, deliberately taken, that hasten death, whilst either relieving suffering or ceasing futile treatment, but this would be grossly unfair, as these are palliative acts of necessity. Physician-assisted dying is just such a palliative act, different in method, but palliative beyond doubt. It is for this reason that I have deliberately refrained from the use of the word 'kill' in relation to voluntary euthanasia or any other death-hastening palliative act. It is no more appropriate to single out voluntary euthanasia by lethal injection or 'assisted suicide' for this description than other palliative acts. The only valid distinction is that voluntary euthanasia by lethal injection hastens death abruptly, whereas other palliative acts hasten death by hours or days.

The inadequacy of the criminal law in this area is emphasised by the respected counsel Richard McGarvie in the introductory quote to this chapter. David Malcolm, Chief Justice of the WA Supreme Court, expressed a similar view:

> At present members of the medical profession are placed in a very difficult position where they have patients who are terminally ill and suffering great pain and mental anguish or otherwise suffering, who know that matters need to be brought to a dignified end. The dilemma facing doctors are the twin obligations to preserve life and to relieve suffering. Preserving life is increasingly

meaningless when a terminally ill patient is close to death, and the emphasis on relieving suffering becomes a risk to the patient's life. This means that the treatment to relieve pain and suffering which co-incidentally might bring forward the moment of death by a few hours or days is acceptable; the principle of double effect, but administering a drug such as potassium or curare, with the primary intention of causing death is not. The question is should we leave doctors in this exposed situation without statutory protection?[19]

The wise and experienced Palliative Care Professor Michael Ashby made this penetrating comment:

In their criminal codes most societies deem themselves to have an interest in preserving the lives of their citizens which overrides any individual's wishes for medical assistance in dying. This is unacceptable to many people who give the highest priority to personal autonomy and control over their life decisions. There is the potential for alienating these people from mainstream medical services if their views are ignored or rejected in a paternalistic way. Those caring for people making such requests should continue to offer and deliver care without allowing personal religious beliefs to intrude into the clinical encounter.[20]

His equally wise colleague Professor Allan Kellehear had this to say:

As a palliative care professional, I oppose euthanasia as a personal choice, but I support its legislation. I will always try to talk you out of that choice. But if you can stand it no longer I would understand your wish and your act to go. I would support your autonomy because you are a free citizen in a multicultural society, and not the plaything of clinical and religious institutions.[21]

How long must this hypocritical farce continue before some parliament has the courage to defy the wrath of the organised religions and introduce legislation that allows for people with intolerable and unrelievable suffering to choose the means of palliation that they feel is appropriate to their life's values? Physician-assisted dying, by whatever method, is palliative treatment—let people choose what is best for them.

In this book I have described a number of contexts in which requests have been made, and ways in which I have assisted people to end their own lives by their choice. In every case I have acted with the primary intention of palliating their suffering, whilst accepting that it was their intention to hasten their death in order to relieve their intolerable suffering, and acknowledging that my assistance would be highly likely to result in hastening of their death.

The Parliament of Victoria in 1988 was brave enough to say that it recognised the desirability of ensuring that dying patients receive maximum relief of pain and suffering. However, it is apparent in 2008 that the Parliament of the Commonwealth does not have the courage to say how this is to be achieved, how to grant citizens this right without placing their doctor in jeopardy. Perhaps it must be through our courts of justice that a defining decision will be reached. If a court accepts that physician-assisted dying in appropriate circumstances is primarily an act of palliation, then the parliament may become irrelevant in finally helping those with terrible suffering to achieve a good death.

AFTERWORD

How you can choose and achieve a dignified death

Most places in the world, including Victoria and other Australian States, do not have legislation that allows a person with intolerable and unrelievable suffering to request assistance in dying from their doctor. The only places where this is possible are Belgium, the Netherlands, Switzerland and the US state of Oregon.

However, there are many things that people can do in the present circumstance to help someone choose and achieve a dignified death. These things are fundamentally the same wherever you live. Unfortunately, though, many people are totally unaware of them. This postscript is designed to help people understand this process.

Essential inter-related principles
1. Understanding—your disease and the law in relation to dying
2. Preparation—to control your dying
3. Communication—with your doctors and family
4. Acceptance—of the reality of dying

Most states and countries have dying with dignity or voluntary euthanasia organisations that are dedicated to law reform, but are also a fount of information regarding the law and palliative care in their country. They are an excellent starting point for information. In Victoria, that organisation is Dying With Dignity Victoria, 3/9b Salisbury Ave, Blackburn, 3130; telephone 03 9877 7677, fax 03 9877 5077, www.dwdv.org.au, e-mail dwdv@dwdv.org.au.

Understanding the law and your disease
Although laws vary between states and countries, today most have common themes. They will almost certainly give statutory, or at least common law, protection to the right of a fully informed, competent person

to refuse medical treatment. No doctor should be able to impose life-prolonging treatment that you do not want.

Understanding your disease means you should be fully aware of your disease, how it is likely to progress, what complications you might encounter and what treatments are available. Armed with this understanding, you can make fully informed decisions as to what treatment you do or do not want. Your doctors are obliged to provide you with full and frank information if you request it.

Most states or countries will have legislation that allows you to appoint an agent to make medical decisions on your behalf if you become incompetent. This protects your autonomy if you suffer a severe brain condition. It can protect you from having your life prolonged when there is no chance of recovering any ability to think normally and communicate intelligently.

Many states and countries will also have formal Refusal of Treatment certificates that you can complete to prevent unwanted treatment in the event of a serious complication of a current illness. For example, if you suffer from advanced heart or respiratory disease, you may refuse resuscitative treatment for a highly likely future catastrophe such as a massive heart attack, massive stroke or respiratory failure. You can request maximum relief of pain and suffering so that you will not suffer from the refusal of treatment.

Many states and countries also allow you to make an advance directive to place in writing your wishes in the event of your losing the ability to communicate them.

Most states will have an appointed official to assist in resolving disputes regarding treatment (in Victoria, it is the Health Services Commissioner), and a Public Advocate to represent people with disability. If you have a loved one who has not appointed an agent to make decisions, you can apply for the appointment of a guardian.

Preparation to control your dying
This involves obtaining and completing the appropriate forms and having your signature witnessed. They must then be copied and

distributed to anyone who might be involved in your care in the event of a serious illness. This includes your legally appointed agent, your family, your local doctor and any specialists who are treating you, and any hospital or institution that you may attend.

Remember this: if confronted by serious illness, an incompetent patient and no information as to the patient's wishes, the doctor's default position is to treat the patient. If you have reached a point where you do not want any further life-prolonging treatment, you need to make that decision clear and have it documented. Most doctors will be only too grateful to have such clear direction.

Communication with your doctors and family

This is probably the most important principle. Suffering is personal, and another person does not know or necessarily understand the nature or depth of your suffering unless you tell them, firmly and, if necessary, repeatedly. Another person cannot see or measure your pain (unless it is extreme), nor can they see or measure your psychological and existential distress. They can imagine it, feel it, but cannot actually experience another's suffering in this regard. A doctor cannot treat suffering that he or she is unaware of.

You must communicate the nature and extent of any suffering, and if treatment is given but is not sufficient, you must say so.

If you have reached a point where you want maximum relief of pain and suffering, tell your doctor clearly. Doctors are fearful of being accused of excessive or aggressive treatment; they will be reassured by a request for more aggressive treatment coming from a patient and supported by their family.

Do not ask your doctor for euthanasia in the presence of others, although you may ask him or her for maximum relief of pain and suffering. Don't wait for your doctor to bring up this subject—he or she usually will be reluctant, not wanting to create the impression that they are disinterested in your future survival. If you know your doctor well, you could ask him or her for medication to give you control over the end of your life. The result might surprise you.

If you and your family are struggling with your illness, ask about palliative care; or if it is suggested for you, accept it gratefully. Palliative care is probably the most important medical development of the past forty years and is of the utmost benefit to most dying people. Make your wishes clear to the carers, and if they are not meeting your needs, say so.

If you are terminally ill, you will be at one of the weakest points of your life. You need support and strong advocates in seeing that your wishes are met. Your family, and perhaps strong friends, are your most important allies. That is why you must communicate effectively with them about your wishes, about your suffering. You will be communicating, not complaining. They will not want to lose you, but they need to realise that there is a time to let go, and that to persist with futile treatment will only make you suffer more. You may need to be persistent in this communication.

This dialogue with your doctor and your family cannot start too soon, particularly if you are diagnosed with a potentially fatal illness. It is extremely difficult to have an adequate dialogue when a crisis has erupted.

Acceptance of the reality of dying

Some people may have different views on this matter, but my experience is that people die better once they have accepted the reality of dying. Much precious time can be wasted by chasing a miraculous cure or through fighting a battle that cannot be won. False hope can lead to false and harmful investigation and treatment.

> *Do not go gentle into that good night*
> *Rage, rage against the dying of the light*

These words of the great Welsh poet Dylan Thomas are wonderful poetry, but bad advice. Anger, frustration and bitterness are bad companions on life's last journey. It is a time for love, friendship and peace.

NOTES

Preface

1 Bert Keizer, 1996.
2 Timothy Quill, *New England Journal of Medicine*, 1991, p. 691.
3 Walter Kade, *Annals of Internal Medicine*, 2000, p. 504.
4 Eric Cassel, *Annals of Internal Medicine*, 1999, p. 531.

1 Epiphany

1 CS Cleeland confirmed this in his editorial in the *Journal of the American Medical Association*, 1998, p. 1914.
2 American Geriatrics Society, p. 635.
3 MLS Vachon et al., 1995, p. 142.
4 M Ashby, 1995a, p. 152.
5 Catholic Church, 1995.

2 The Journey Begins

1 Declan Walsh, 1993, p. 350.
2 MM Cohen, 1992, p. 317.
3 I Higginson & M McCarthy, 1989, p. 264.
4 L Gibbs et al., 1998, p. 1961.
5 M McCarthy & J Addington-Hall, 1997, p. 128.
6 M Angell, 1999, p. 1923.
7 ibid.
8 Council of Judicial and Ethical Affairs, 1992b, p. 2229.
9 Australian Medical Association, 2002.
10 Jenny Uglow, 2002, p. 463.
11 CD Douglas et al., 2001, p. 511.
12 T Quill, 1993, p. 1039.
13 P Ariès, 1981.

3 Defining the Problem

1 D Meier, 1997, p. 225.
2 SB Nuland, 1993.
3 Ivan Illich, 1975.

4   R Fainsinger et al., 2000, p. 257.

5   J Lynn et al., 1997, p. 106.

6   K Faber-Langenden & PN Lanken, 2000, p. 886.

7   Ivan Lichter & Esther Hunt, 1990, p. 7.

8   Declan Walsh, 1993, p. 350.

9   Erich Loewy, 2001, p. 329.

10   D Martin et al., 2000, p. 1672.

11   MP Battin, 1994b.

12   Criminal Court Ruling, *Leeuwarden*, 1973: 'the Postma case'.

13   PJ van der Maas et al., 1991, p. 669.

14   FG Miller, 1998, p. 138.

15   World Medical Association, 39th World Medical Assembly, Madrid, 1987.

16   House of Lords (session 1993–1994), *Report of the Select Committee on Medical Ethics*, Volume 1, Report, p. 11, para 26.

17   Catholic Church, Pope John Paul II, 1995, para. 65.

18   S Chater, 1998, p. 255.

19   Aycke Smook, personal communication to author, The World Federation of Right to Die Societies conference, Toronto, 2006.

20   Charles McKhann, 1999.

21   Newspoll 2007; Roy Morgan Research, 2002 (Australia); Gallup Poll, 2006; AP-Ipsos Poll, 2007 (USA); A-P Ipsos poll, 2007 (Canada); Massey University, 2003 (NZ).

22   John Zalcberg, 1996.

5 A Hot Potato

1   H Kuhse & P Singer, 1992, p. 21.

2   Rodney Syme, 1991, p. 203.

3   M Ragg, 1992.

6 Crossing the Line

1   T Quill, 1991, p. 691.

2   ibid.

3 J Addington-Hall & L Kalra, 2001.
4 Clive Seale & Julia Addington-Hall, 1994, p. 647.
5 Erich Loewy, 2001, p. 329.

7 Prolonging Life

1 Nick Davies, 1995.
2 Reprinted, unedited, with permission.
3 Nessa Coyle et al., 1990, p. 83.
4 Roger Hunt et al., 1995, p. 167.
5 Clive Seale & Julia Addington-Hall, 1995, p. 581.

8 The Nature of Suffering

1 Walter Kade, 2000, p. 504.

9 Terminal Sedation

1 Jessica Corner, 1997, p. 1242.
2 Ivan Lichter & Esther Hunt, 1990, p. 7.
3 E De Sousa & B Jepson, 1988.
4 V Ventafridda et al., 1990, p. 7.
5 DM Bottomly & GW Hanks, 1990, p. 259.
6 AL Burke et al., 1991, p. 485.
7 N Cherny et al., 1994, p. 71.
8 M Ashby, 1995a, p. 152.
9 Alan Fleischman, 1998, p. 138.

10 Respecting Choice

1 Ronald Dworkin, 1993.
2 Jean-Dominique Bauby, 1997.
3 L Darvall et al., 2001, p. 167.
4 Council of Judicial and Ethical Affairs, 1992a, pp. 18–19.
5 JL Bernat, 1994, p. 372.
6 ibid., p. 347.
7 *Cruzan v. Director, Missouri Department of Health*, 497 US 288–90, O'Connor, J.
8 Ivan Illich, 1975.

9   William Colby, 2006.

10 J Ahronheim et al., 1996, p. 2094.

11 Ivan Illich, 1995, p. 1652.

12 Mukesh Haikerwal, as cited in G Costa, 2002.

13 B Pollard, 1991, p. 559.

14 *Gardner, re BWV*, [2003] JVSC 173.

15 M Ashby, 2002.

16 P Howard, 1999.

17 *Airedale NHS Trust v. Bland*, [199] AC 789.

18 ibid.

19 ibid.

20 J Kassubek et al., 2003, p. 85.

21 ibid.

11 A Difficult Situation

1   T Quill, 1997, p. 2099.

2   H Kuhse & P Singer, 1988, p. 623; P Baume & E O'Malley, p. 137;
    M Steinberg et al., 1997, p. 131; D Neil et al., 2007, p. 721.

3   Neil MacDonald et al., 1995, p. 151.

4   Charles McKhann, 1999.

12 A Reportable Death?

1   N Cherny et al., 1996, p. 261.

2   V Ventafridda et al., 1990, p. 7.

3   RG Twycross, 1993, pp. 651–61.

4   David J Roy, 1990, p. 3.

13 Is This the Best We Can Do?

1   D Martin et al., 2000, p. 1672.

2   M Levy, 1996, p. 1124.

3   M Ashby, 1995b, p. 596.

4   M Ashby, 1995a, p. 152.

5   R Hunt, 1994.

6   M Albom, 1997.

7   Darren Gray, 1999.

8   Linda Emanuel, 1998, p. 643.
9   B Gert et al., 1998.
10 N Cherny et al., 1996. p. 261.
11 JL Bernat, 1993, p. 2723.
12 Parliament of Victoria, 1986, p. 106.
13 N Tonti-Filipini, 1992, p. 277.
14 Rodney Syme, 1999.

14 Provoking the Coroner

1   Erich Loewy, 2001, p. 329.
2   E Bruera et al., 1992, p. 192.
3   JL Bernat, 1994.
4   Ellen McGee, 1997, p. 27.
5   Misha Ketchell, 2001.
6   Palliative Care Australia, 1999.
7   HM Chochinov et al., 2005, p. 5520.
8   Ellen McGee, 1997, p. 27.
9   Derek Doyle, 1992, p. 302.
10 Donna Casey, 2007.
11 M Ashby, 1995b, p. 596.
12 P Ravenscroft, as cited in R Ecclestone, 1997.
13 Janet Hardy, 2000, p. 1866.
14 Linda Emanuel, 1998, p. 643.
15 J Luce & J Luce, 2001, p. 1131.
16 Erich Loewy, 2001, p. 329.
17 Jonathon Glover, 1977, p. 287.
18 Mukesh Haikerwal, as cited in G Costa, 2002.
19 CS Cleeland, 1998, p. 1914.
20 P Kempen, 1999, p. 605.
21 B McDonald, as cited in *Victorian Senior*, 2007.
22 J Bernheim et al., 2008.
23 E Emanuel, 2003, p. 203.
24 M Ashby, 1995b, p. 596.
25 K Rayner, 1993.
26 John Zalcberg, 1996.

27 Ian Maddocks, *Science Show*, radio program, ABC Radio, 13 April 1996.
28 J Zalcberg & J Buchanan, 1997, p. 150.
29 Stanley Terman, 2007.

15 Fear of the Future

1 PA Singer et al., 1999, p. 163.
2 Palliative Care Australia, 2004.
3 Barbara Fiveash, 1997.
4 Allan Kellehear & David Ritchie (eds), 2003.
5 Eric Cassell, 1999, p. 531.
6 PA Singer et al., 1999, p. 163.
7 Peter Hudson et al., 2006, p. 693.
8 MP Battin, 1994a, p. 175.
9 American Academy of Hospice and Palliative Medicine, 2007.
10 T Quill, 2007, p. 1911.
11 L Minelli, personal communication, 23 April 2007.
12 I Haverkate et al., 2000, p. 865.
13 Kate Legge, 2005.

16 A Good Death: Jim Dies in His Own Bed

1 M Barbato, 1998, p. 296.
2 *Cruzan v. Director, Missouri Department of Health*, 497 US 261 (1990).
3 Linda Ganzini, 1998, p. 967.
4 Martin Klein, 2004, p. 225.
5 Oregon Department of Human Services, 2007.
6 Daniel Lee, 2003, pp. 17–19.
7 Janet Hardy, 2000, p. 1866.
8 LC Kaldjian et al., 2004, p. 499.
9 *R v. Davidson*, [1969] VR 667, Supreme Court of Victoria, Menhennitt, J.

17 The Suffering Mind

1 Andrew Solomon, 2002.
2 Anne Deveson, 1998.

3   Mary Jane Massie et al., 1994, p. 325.

4   N Shah, 1998, p. 352.

5   HM Chochinov, 1997, p. 67.

18 Regaining Control

1   Palliative Care Australia, 2007.

2   W Breitbart et al., 2000, p. 2907.

3   Marcia Angell, 2004.

4   ibid.

5   M Ashby, 1995b, p. 596.

19 Steve Guest: A Death Not in Vain

1   Steve Guest is the real name of the man I treat in this chapter (unlike all other chapters). John Guest is his brother. Their names are used with their full consent.

2   David J Roy, 1990, p. 3.

3   N MacDonald et al., 1995, p. 151.

4   S Morrison & D Meier, 2004, p. 2585.

5   N Coyle et al., 1990, p. 83.

6   H Chochinov, 2002, p. 2253.

7   Julie Anne Davies, 2007.

8   David Lanham, 1992.

9   Ellen McGee, 1997, p. 27.

10 M Barbato, 1998, p. 296.

11 NI Cherny et al., 1994, p. 71.

12 D Neil et al., 2007, p. 721.

13 Roger Magnussen, 2002.

14 Loane Skene, 2003.

15 M Otlowski, 1993, p. 10.

16 ibid.

20 Dying With Dignity

1   Tessa Richards, 2007, p. 830.

2   Palliative Care Australia, 2007.

3   Peter Hudson et al., 2006, p. 693.

4   Linda Emanuel, 1998, p. 643.
5   Rodney Syme, 1987.
6   David Asch, 1998, p. 135.
7   J Billings & S Block, 1996, p. 21.
8   Roger Magnussen, 2002.
9   M Ashby, 1995b, p. 596.
10 D Fishbein, 1989, p. 76.
11 MM Cohen, 1992, p. 317.
12 RG Twycross, 1996, p. 61.
13 M Ashby, 1995b, p. 596.
14 D Neil et al., 2007, p. 721.
15 T Quill, 2004, p. 2029.
16 N Christakis & P Allison, 2006, p. 719.
17 Polly Toynbee, 2004.
18 Kenny Goldberg, 2007.
19 David Malcolm, 1998, p. 46.
20 M Ashby, 1995b, p. 596.
21 A Kellehear, 2003.

BIBLIOGRAPHY

Books

Albom, M, *Tuesdays with Morrie*, Doubleday, Westminster, MD, 1997.

Angell, Marcia, 'The Quality of Mercy', in TE Quill & MP Battin (eds), *Physician Assisted Dying*, The Johns Hopkins University Press, Baltimore, MD, 2004.

Ariès, P, *The Hour of Our Death*, Oxford University Press, 1981.

Battin, MP, *Ethical Issues in Suicide*, Prentice-Hall, Engelwood Cliffs, NJ, 1994a.

—— *Least Worst Death*, Oxford University Press, 1994b.

Bauby, Jean-Dominique, *The Diving-Bell and the Butterfly*, Fourth Estate, London, 1997.

Bernat, JL, *Ethical Issues in Neurology*, Butterworth-Heinemann, Boston, 1994.

Colby, William, *Unplugged: Reclaiming our right to die in America*, AMACOM, New York, 2007.

Deveson, Anne, *Tell Me I'm Here*, 2nd edn, Penguin, Camberwell, VIC, 1998.

Dworkin, Ronald, *Life's Dominion*, Knopf, New York, 1993.

Glover, Jonathon, *Causing Death and Saving Lives*, Penguin, Harmondsworth, 1977.

Hunt, R, *Willing to Listen, Wanting to Die*, Penguin Books, Ringwood, Vic, 1994.

Illich, Ivan, *Medical Nemesis*, Calder and Byers, London, 1975.

Keizer, Bert, *Dancing with Mister D: notes on life and death*, Doubleday, London, 1996.

Kellehear, Allan, & David Ritchie (eds), *Seven Dying Australians*, Innovative Resources, Bendigo, Vic, 2003.

Lanham, David, *Taming Death by Law*, Longman Professional, Melbourne, 1992.

Magnussen, Roger, *Angels of Death*, Melbourne University Press, Carlton, 2002.

McKhann, Charles, *A Time to Die*, Yale University Press, New Haven, 1999.

Nuland, SB, *How We Die*, Chatto and Windus, London, 1993.

Skene, Loane, *Law and Medical Practice: Rights, duties, claims and defences*, LexisNexis Butterworths, Sydney, 2003.

Solomon, Andrew, *The Noonday Demon: An anatomy of depression*, Vintage, Westminster, MD, 2002.

Terman, Stanley, *The Best Way to Say Goodbye: A legal peaceful choice at the end of life*, Life Transitions Publications, Carlsbad, CA, 2007.

Twycross, RG, *Oxford Textbook of Palliative Medicine*, 3rd edn., Oxford University Press, Oxford, 2004.

Uglow, Jenny, *The Lunar Men: Five friends whose curiosity changes the world*, Farrer, Straus & Giraux, New York, 2002.

Journal Articles

Addington-Hall, J, & L Kalra, 'Who should measure quality of life?', *British Medical Journal*, 2001: 332; 1417.

Ahronheim, J, et al., 'Treatment of the dying in the acute care hospital', *Archives of Internal Medicine*, 1996: 156; 2094.

American Geriatrics Society, 'Guidelines', *Journal of the American Geriatrics Society*, 1998: 46; 635.

Angell, M, 'Caring for the dying—congressional mischief', *New England Journal of Medicine*, 1999: 341; 1923.

Asch, David, 'Tensions between theory and practice in palliative care', *Journal of Pain and Symptom Management*, 1998: 16; 135.

Ashby, M, 'Hard cases, causation and care of the dying', *Journal of Law and Medicine*, 1995a: 3; 152.

—— 'The euthanasia controversy. Decision-making in extreme cases', *Medical Journal of Australia*, 1995b: 162; 596.

Barbato, M, 'Death is a journey to be undertaken', *Medical Journal of Australia*, 1998: 168; 296.

Baume, P, & E O'Malley, 'Euthanasia: attitudes and practices of medical practitioners', *Medical Journal of Australia*, 1994: 161; 137.

Bernat, JL, 'Patient refusal of hydration and nutrition', *Archives of Internal Medicine*, 1993: 153; 2723.

Bernheim, JL, et al., 'Development of palliative care and legislation of euthanasia: antagonism or synergy?', *British Medical Journal*, 2008 (at press).

Billings, J, & S Block, 'Slow euthanasia', *Journal of Palliative Care*, 1996: 12; 21.

Bottomly, DM, & GW Hanks, 'Subcutaneous midazolam infusion in palliative care', *Journal of Pain and Symptom Management*, 1990: 5; 259.

Breitbart, W, et al., 'Depression, hopelessness, and the desire for hasteneed death in terminally ill patients with cancer', *Journal of the American Medical Association*, 2000: 284; 2907.

Bruera, E, et al., 'Cognitive failure in patients with terminal cancer: a prospective study', *Journal of Pain and Symptom Management*, 1992: 7; 192.

Burke, AL, et al., 'Terminal restlessness—its management and the role of midazolam', *Medical Journal of Australia*, 1991: 155; 485.

Cassell, Eric, 'Diagnosing suffering: a perspective', *Annals of Internal Medicine*, 1999: 131; 531.

Chater, S, 'Sedation for intractable distress in the dying—a survey of experts', *Palliative Medicine*, 1998: 12; 255.

Cherny, N, et al., 'Guidelines in the care of the dying cancer patient', *Haematology/Oncology Clinics of North America*, 1996: 10; 261.

Cherny, NI, et al., 'The treatment of suffering when patients request elective death', *Journal of Palliative Care*, 1994: 10; 71.

Chochinov, H, 'Dignity-conserving care—a new model for palliative care', *Journal of the American Medical Association*, 2002: 287; 2253.

Chochinov, HM, '"Are you depressed?" Screening for depression in the terminally ill', *American Journal of Psychiatry*, 1997: 154; 67.

Chochinov, HM, et al., 'Dignity therapy: a novel psychotherapeutic intervention for patients near the end of life', *Journal of Clinical Oncology*, 2005: 23; 5520.

Christakis, N, & P Allison, 'Mortality after the hospitalisation of a spouse', *New England Journal of Medicine*, 2006: 354; 719.

Cleeland, CS, Editorial, 'Under treatment of cancer pain in elderly patients', *Journal of the American Medical Association*, 1998: 279; 1914.

Cohen, MM, 'Treatment of intractable dyspnoea: clinical and ethical issues', *Cancer Investigation*, 1992: 10; 317.

Corner, Jessica, 'More openness needed in palliative care', *British Medical Journal*, 1997: 315; 1242.

Council of Judicial and Ethical Affairs, American Medical Association, 'Decisions near the end of life', *Journal of the American Medical Association*, 1992: 267; 2229.

Coyle, N, et al., 'Character of terminal illness in the advanced cancer patient: pain and other symptoms during the last four weeks of life', *Journal of Pain and Symptom Management*, 1990: 5; 83.

Darvall, L, et al., 'Medico-legal knowledge of general practitioners: disjunctions, errors and uncertainties', *Journal of Law and Medicine*, 2001: 9; 167.

De Sousa, E, & B Jepson, 'Midazolam in terminal care', *The Lancet*, 1988: 1; 67.

Douglas, CD, et al., 'The intention to hasten death: a survey of attitudes and practices of surgeons in Australia', *Medical Journal of Australia*, 2001: 175; 511.

Doyle, Derek, 'Have we looked beyond the physical and psychosocial?', *Journal of Pain and Symptom Management*, 1992: 7; 302.

Ecclestone, Roy, 'The consumer's guide to palliative care', *The Australian Magazine*, 15–16 February 1997.

Emanuel, E, (review of Herbert Hendin & Kathleen Foley, *The Case against Assisted Suicide: Or the right to end-of-life care*, Johns Hopkins University Press, Baltimore, 2002), *Journal of the American Medical Association*, 2003: 289; 203.

Emanuel, Linda, 'Facing requests for physician-assisted suicide', *Journal of the American Medical Association*, 1998: 280; 643.

Faber-Langenden, K, & PN Lanken, 'Dying patients in the intensive care unit', *Annals of Internal Medicine*, 2000: 138; 886.

Fainsinger, R, et al., 'A multi-centre international study of sedation for uncontrolled symptoms in terminally ill patients', *Palliative Medicine*, 2000: 14; 257.

Fishbein, D, 'An approach to dyspnoea in cancer patients', *Journal of Pain and Symptom Management*, 1989: 4; 76.

Fleischman, Alan, 'Ethical issues in paediatric pain management and terminal sedation', *Journal of Pain and Symptom Management*, 1998: 15; 138.

Ganzini, Linda, 'Attitudes of patients with ALS (motor neurone disease) and their care givers towards assisted suicide', *New England Journal of Medicine*, 1998: 339; 967.

Gert, B, et al., 'An alternative to physician assisted suicide', in MP Battin (ed.), *Physician Assisted Suicide—Expanding the Debate,* Routledge, London, 1998.

Gibbs, L, et al., 'Dying from heart failure: lessons from palliative care', *British Medical Journal,* 1998: 317; 1961.

Goldberg, Kenny, 'Leading hospice organization drops opposition to doctor-assisted suicide', KPBS News, San Diego State University, CA, 28 Feburary 2007.

Hardy, Janet, 'Sedation in terminally ill patients', *The Lancet,* 2000: 356; 1866.

Haverkate, I, et al., 'Refused and granted requests for euthanasia and assisted suicide in the Netherlands', *British Medical Journal,* 2000: 321; 865.

Higginson, I, & M McCarthy, 'Measuring symptoms in terminal cancer: are pain and dyspnoea controlled?', *Proceedings of the Royal Society of Medicine,* 1989: 82; 264.

Hudson, Peter, et al., 'Desire for hastened death in patients with advanced disease and the evidence base of clinical guidelines: a systematic review', *Palliative Medicine,* 2006: 20; 693.

Hunt, Roger, et al., 'The incidence of requests for a quicker terminal course', *Palliative Medicine,* 1995: 9; 167.

Illich, Ivan, 'Death undefeated', *British Medical Journal,* 1995: 311; 1652.

Kade, Walter, 'Death with dignity—a case study', *Annals of Internal Medicine,* 2000: 132; 504.

Kaldjian, LC, et al., 'Internists attitudes towards terminal sedation in end of life care', *Journal of Medical Ethics,* 2004: 30; 499.

Kassubek, J, et al., 'Activation of a risidual cortical network during painful stimulation in long-term postanoxic vegetative state', *Journal of Neurological Science,* 2003: 15; 85.

Kempen, P, 'Managing pain in elderly patients', *Journal of the American Medical Association,* 1999: 281; 605.

Klein, Martin, 'Voluntary euthanasia and the doctrine of double effect', *Health Care Analysis,* 2004: 12; 225.

Kuhse, H, & P Singer, 'Doctors' practices and attitudes regarding voluntary euthanasia', *Medical Journal of Australia,* 1988: 148; 623.

—— 'Euthanasia: A survey of nurses' attitudes and practices', *Australian Nurses Journal*, 1992: 21; 21.

Lee, Daniel, 'Physician assisted suicide: a conservative critique of intervention', *Hastings Centre Report*, 33, no. 1, 2003, pp. 17–19.

Levy, M, 'Pharmacologic treatment of cancer pain', *New England Journal of Medicine*, 1996: 335; 1124.

Lichter, Ivan, & Esther Hunt, 'The last 48 hours of life', *Journal of Palliative Care*, 1990: 6(4); 7.

Loewy, Erich, 'Terminal sedation, self-starvation, and orchestrating the end of life', *Archives of Internal Medicine*, 2001: 161; 329.

Luce, J, & J Luce, 'Management of dyspnoea in patients with far advanced lung disease', *Journal of the American Medical Association*, 2001: 285; 1131.

Lynn, J, et al., 'US SUPPORT Study', *Annals of Internal Medicine*, 1997: 126; 106.

MacDonald, Neil, et al., 'Cachexia-anorexia-asthenia', *Journal of Pain and Symptom Management*, 1995: 10; 151.

Malcolm, David, 'Euthanasia and the law', *ANZ Medical Journal*, 1998: 28; 46.

Martin, D, et al., 'Planning for the end of life', *The Lancet*, 2000: 356; 1672.

Massie, Mary Jane, et al., 'Depression and suicide in patients with cancer', *Journal of Pain and Symptom Management*, 1994: 9; 325.

McCarthy, M, & J Addington-Hall, 'Communication and choice in dying from heart disease', *Journal of Pain and Symptom Management*, 1997: 19; 128.

McGee, Ellen, 'Can suicide intervention in hospice be ethical', *Journal of Palliative Care*, 1997: 13; 27.

Meier, D, et al., 'Improving palliative care', *Annals of Internal Medicine*, 1997: 127; 225.

Miller, FG, 'Professional integrity in the home', *Journal of Pain and Symptom Management*, 1998: 15; 138.

Morrison, S, & D Meier, 'Palliative care', *New England Journal of Medicine*, 2004: 350; 2585.

Neil, D, et al., 'End-of-life decisions in medical practice; a survey of doctors in Victoria (Australia)', *Journal of Medical Ethics*, 2007: 33; 721.

Otlowski, M, 'Mercy killing cases in the Australian criminal justice system', *Criminal Law Journal*, 1993: 17; 10.

Pollard, B, 'Withdrawing life-sustaining treatment from severely brain-damaged persons', *Medical Journal of Australia*, 1991: 154; 559.

Quill, T, 'Death and dignity: a case of individualized decision making', *New England Journal of Medicine*, 1991: 324; 691.

—— 'The ambiguity of clinical intentions', *Journal of the American Medical Association*, 1993: 329; 1039.

—— 'Palliative options of last resort', *Journal of the American Medical Association*, 1997: 278; 2099.

—— 'Dying and decision making—evolution of end-of-life options', *New England Journal of Medicine*, 2004: 350; 2029.

—— 'Legal regulation of physician-assisted death—the latest report card', *New England Journal of Medicine*, 2007: 356; 1911.

Ragg, M, 'Australia: for or against euthanasia?', *The Lancet*, 1992: 339; 800.

Rayner, K, William Arnold Connolly Oration to the Royal Australian College of General Practitioners, *Australian Family Physician,* 1993: 22; 545.

Richards, Tessa, 'A better way to die', *British Medical Journal*, 2007: 334; 830.

Roy, David J, 'Need they sleep before they die?', *Journal of Palliative Care*, 1990: 6; 3.

Seale, Clive, & Julia Addington-Hall, 'Euthanasia: the role of good care, *Social Science Medicine*', 1995: 40; 581.

—— 'Euthanasia: why people want to die earlier', *Social Science Medicine*, 1994: 39; 647.

Shah, N, 'National survey of UK psychiatrists' attitudes to euthanasia', *The Lancet*, 1998: 352.

Singer, PA, et al., 'Quality end-of-life care: patients' perspectives', *Journal of the American Medical Association*, 1999; 281: 163.

Steinberg, M, et al., 'End-of-life decision-making: community and medical practitioners' perspectives', *Medical Journal of Australia*, 1997: 166; 131.

Syme, Rodney, 'A patient's right to a good death', *Medical Journal of Australia*, 1991: 154; 203.

Tonti-Filipini, N, 'Some refusals of medical treatment which changed the law of Victoria', *Medical Journal of Australia*, 1992: 157; 277.

Toynbee, Polly, *Guardian Unlimited*, 10 December 2004.

Twycross, RG, 'Euthanasia: Going Dutch?', *Journal of the Royal Society of Medicine*, 1996: 89; 61.

Vachon, MLS, et al., 'Psychosocial issues in palliative care: the patient, the family and the process and outcome of care', *Journal of Pain and Symptom Management*, 1995: 10; 142.

van der Maas, PJ, et al., 'Euthanasia and other medical decisions concerning the end of life', *The Lancet*, 1991: 338; 669.

Ventafridda, V, et al., 'Symptom prevalence and control during cancer patients' last days of life', *Journal of Palliative Care*, 1990: 6(3); 7.

Walsh, Declan, 'Dyspnoea in advanced cancer', *The Lancet*, 1993: 342; 450.

Zalcberg, J, & J Buchanan, 'Clinical issues in euthanasia', *Medical Journal of Australia*, 1997: 166; 150.

Newspapers

Casey, Donna, 'Patients push debate', *Ottawa Sun*, 7 November 2007.

Costa, Gabrielle, 'Litigation fears over dying patient', *The Age*, 16 July 2002.

Davies, Julie Anne, 'Terminal answer', *The Bulletin*, 6 November 2007.

Davies, Nick, 'Helping patients to die (Melbourne Seven)', *The Age*, 25 March 1995.

Gray, Darren, 'Two faces of debate on right to die', *The Age*, 14 April 1999.

Howard, P, letter, *The Times*, 28 June 1999.

Kaszubska, Gosia, 'Right to life case critical', *The Australian*, 24 December 2002.

Ketchell, Misha, 'Loophole for lethal drug use claimed', *The Age*, 21 June 2000.

Legge, Kate, 'Choosing one's time to go', *The Australian*, 12 February 2005.

Syme, Rodney, 'Dying without dignity', *The Age*, 31 August 1999.

—— letter, *The Age*, 23 June 1987.

Victorian Senior, 9 September 2007.

Zalcberg, John, 'Symptom control, palliative care or euthanasia?', *Medical Observer*, 19 January 1996.

Cases

Airedale NHS Trust v. Bland, [199] AC 789.

Criminal Court Ruling, *Leeuwarden*, 1973: 'the Postma case', Netherlands.

Cruzan v. Director, Missouri Department of Health, 497 US, 1990, (O'Connor, J).
Gardner, re BWV, [2003] JVSC 173.
R v. Davidson, [1969] VR 667, Supreme Court of Victoria, Menhennitt, J.

Legislation

Consent to Medical Treatment and Palliative Care Act 1995 (SA)
Coroners Act 1985 (Vic)
Crimes Act 1958 (Vic)
Death with Dignity Act 1997 (Oregon, USA)
Medical Treatment Act 1988 (Vic)

Other

American Academy of Hospice and Palliative Medicine, 'Physician-assisted Death', Position statement, Glenview, IL, 14 February 2007.
AP-Ipsos Poll, 2007 (Canada).
AP-Ipsos Poll, 2007 (USA).
Australian Medical Association, AMA Federal Assembly, May 2002.
Catholic Church, *The Charter for Health Care Workers*, Vatican, Vatican City, 1995.
Catholic Church, Pope John Paul II, *Evangelium vitae (the gospel of life) to the bishops, priests and deacons, men and women religious lay faithful and all people of good will on the value and inviolability of human life*, Vatican, Vatican City, 25 March 1995.
Fiveash, Barbara, *Lincoln Papers in Gerontology*, No 36, Latrobe University, Melbourne, 1997.
Gallup Poll, 2006.
House of Lords (session 1993–1994), *Report of the Select Committee on Medical Ethics, Volume 1, Report*.
Kellehear, A, Address to Voluntary Euthanasia Society of Victoria, Melbourne, 2003.
Newspoll, 2007.
Roy Morgan Research, 2002 (Australia).
Massey University, 2003 (NZ).
Oregon Department of Human Services, *Ninth Annual Report on Oregon's Death with Dignity Act*, Portland, OR, 6 March 2007.

Palliative Care Australia, Position Statement on Euthanasia, Deakin, ACT, 1999.

—— *The Hardest Thing We Have Ever Done—The Social Impact of Caring for Terminally Ill People in Australia: Full Report of the National Inquiry into the Social Impact of Caring for Terminally Ill People*, prepared by Samar Aoun, Palliative Care Australia, Deakin, ACT, 2004.

—— 'Dying choices—far more than a one-issue debate', media release, Deakin, ACT, 1 February 2007.

Parliament of Victoria, Social Development Committee, *Inquiry into Options for Dying with Dignity, Second and Final Report*, 1986.

World Medical Association, 39th World Medical Assembly, Madrid, 1987.

INDEX

sense of burden, 184–5, 186
Seven Dying Australians, 187
Shah, Dr Nisha, 222
Singer, Professor Peter, 42, 143, 254
Skene, Professor Loane, 247–8
Smook, Dr Aycke, xvii, 28, 211
Stephens, Dr Daryl, 240, 247
stroke, 19, 53, 86–7, 107–8, 112, 172, 186, 189, 192, 256, 273
suicide; assisted, 52–3, 268; in common law, 159–60; *Crimes Act* on, 40; failed, 51–2; fear of implicating family, 52; irrational, 31–2; a last resort, 7; meaning, 31; in older people, 267; rational, 32; seen as an option, 236; stigma of, 193–4
Susan, 224–7, 256
Switzerland, 195, 219, 272
Syme, Rodney; advocates law change, 43; *The Age* article, 43, 49; and article by Quill, 46–7; defines voluntary euthanasia, 29–31; enters euthanasia debate, 253–4; explores terminal sedation, 254–5; fear of discovery, 50, 233; first press interview, 43; implications from reported cases, 169–70; impossible to solve everyone's problems, 218; looks for alternative, 170; when not the treating doctor, 268; philosophy of end-of-life care, 261–5; Ragg article on, 44; realises people's rights to end suffering, 7–8; reputation as doctor who would discuss problem, 43; respects right to self-determination, 43, 63; researches best practice, 142; seeks clarification of own position, 133; spokesman for Dying With Dignity, 228; test case decision, 240
Syme journey of discovery; assistance in absence of depression (Knight), 254; consults the coroner over reportable deaths, 132–3, 139–42; crosses Rubicon by hastening death (Ken), 11, 14; effective medical assistance (Jim, Victor), 256; 'epiphany' (Betty), 1–7, 253; exposure to prosecution

(Margaret), 254; family involved in instructions (Jim), 202–4; first deliberate assistance in dying (Alice), 49–59, 61; first explicit request (Alice), 49–50; first palliation that hastens death (Ken), 10–13; first referrals from doctors and requests from patients, 45; first responsibility for terminally ill patient (Betty), 1–7, 253; first uses terminal sedation as a primary treatment (Pamela), 138–9; helping, but not treating doctor (Alice), 53–4, 56, 61; legal ramifications of care (Harold), 110–12; medication dosage problem, 39, 60; moving beyond helping (Helen), 189, 191–2; obtaining effective medication (Alice), 254; oral prescription best way to assist, 43; patient 'bails out' of commitment (Keith), 123–31; problems of covert practice (Keith), 130–1; providing dialogue and advice, not medication (Knight), 62–80; questioned by police (Steve Guest), 242; role clarified: to give back control and enhance quality of life (Susan), 227; strangers request help (Alice, Knight, Margaret), 254; terminal dehydration and its palliation (Jane), 150; test case (Steve Guest), 240

Tell Me I'm Here, 218
Terman, Dr Stan, 181–2
terminal dehydration with palliation, 83, 116–17, 118, 181; chance to say goodbye, 139, 142; concept, 149–50; coroner's report, 155–9; doctors confident to use, 133; fear of, 174; hastening death, 176; in not all situations, 229; stress on family, 153; Syme seeks alternative, 170; time to take effect, 153–4
terminal illness; cardiac and respiratory conditions, 10–13, 18; communicating with family, 275; compared with hopeless illness, 144–5; crescendo of